PRAISE FOR *THE SACRIFICES OF SUPERWOMEN*

"As little girls, we are told that we stand on 'steely shoulders'—the shoulders of strong, faithful, and courageous women who looked out for everyone in order to survive. In Dr. Andrea D. Sullivan's new book, *The Sacrifices of Superwomen: Natural Remedies to Restore Balance*, she reminds us that we have grown 'sick and tired of being sick and tired.' Too many Black women are on the front lines saving everyone but themselves. They're super-givers who neglect themselves. Oh, they see their doctors, but they don't really get better. Dr. Sullivan believes that to save our community and our country, we have to save ourselves. Drawing on thirty-seven years of practice as a naturopathic physician, she knows the stresses and problems that Black women face and the health issues we must confront. *Sacrifices* is more than a self-help 'practical tool kit'; it's about charting a new narrative to save ourselves in order to save our nation."

—Donna Brazile, Former Acting Chair of Democratic National Committee, Political Strategist, ABC News Political Analyst, Author, Syndicated Columnist, and Adjunct Assistant Professor at Georgetown University

"*The Sacrifices of Superwomen: Natural Remedies to Restore Balance* by Dr. Andrea Sullivan combines medical, historical, and sociological scholarly research with spiritual/health advice and memoir. The book details the appalling statistics of discrepant health care along racial and gender lines in the United States, delineates the powerful difference in practice and philosophy between naturopathic (including herbal and homeopathic) and allopathic medicine, provides detailed advice for self-directed health care, and introduces the reader to amazing superwomen (most notably, the author herself). You cannot come away from reading Sullivan's treatise unchanged. There is such a wealth of information included that it could best become a resource book rather than a quick read. I recommend the book in the highest possible terms."

—R. Barbara Gitenstein, President Emerita, the College of New Jersey, Senior Consultant and Senior Fellow, Association of Governing Boards (AGB), Author of *Experience Is the Angled Road: Memoir of an Academic*

"Put down your superwoman cape and read this origin story to free yourself from a life of over-sacrificing. If you pick up this book you will not put it down. Your life, your mindless habit, and real solutions are in there. Dr. Andrea Sullivan is a national treasure. She has been preaching the gospel of a naturally healthy lifestyle for over four decades. The chapters on water and sleep alone make her book a true lifesaver. I give advice for a living, but Dr. Sullivan's advice will save your life. Enough of the gimmicks; this is the remedy you need for a happy, healthy, full life."

—Kim Keenan, President of the International Women's Forum of DC and Co-chair of the Internet Innovation Alliance, Former President of the National Bar Association and the District of Columbia Bar, Former longest-serving General Counsel of the National Association for the Advancement of Colored People (NAACP)

"Dr. Andrea Sullivan has written about a topic critically important to the health and well-being of Black women. Drawing on her years of experience and expertise as a naturopathic physician, Dr. Sullivan skillfully crafts the persona of the superwoman and brings to light compelling and thought-provoking issues that resonate with Black women of all ages and across all socioeconomic strata.

"Her depiction of superwomen draws upon case examples from her work. She highlights the all-too-familiar stories of selflessness and sacrifice characteristic of women who have internalized oppression and who may have unresolved personal issues that stem from childhood. Indeed, for Black women, the historical narratives of our ancestors who endured tremendous hardship and bore the weight of their people to achieve elusive freedom is ingrained in our psyche, even today. We unwittingly take on the mantle of heroes like Sojourner Truth and Harriet Tubman to the detriment of our own health.

"By boldly telling her own story, Dr. Sullivan shines a light on these internalized narratives and underscores the critical importance of understanding the long-term physical health impacts and the psychological sequelae stemming from adverse childhood experiences and historical trauma. She thoughtfully explains the role of the naturopathic physician and her unique role in helping to promote well-being, including positive affect, physical, and physiologic well-being and the conscious alignment of mind and body in the well care of her patients.

"A key theme in this volume is the focus on stress. Dr. Sullivan unpacks the literal denotation of the word 'stress' as well as the collateral effects and damage of such stressors as sexism and racism. She explains in layman's terms how the immune system works and what we need to do with the help of homeopathic medicine to have our system work at optimal levels. The notion that inflammation and stress are the basis of most disease is both compelling and encouraging in that, as Dr. Sullivan noted, they are understandable, preventable, and treatable. Good health is in our own hands.

"Dr. Sullivan skillfully weaves together a remedy for disease using powerful affirmations throughout the book that help the reader to value themselves and remind them of their self-worth. She concludes with her story and offers simple, everyday steps to help us slowly remove our superwoman cloak, and to don the immutable cape of our inner superpower—self-love.

"I AM LOVED. I AM WELL. I AM GOD'S CHILD."

—Valerie Maholmes, PhD, CAS, Chief, Pediatric Trauma and Clinical Illness Branch, Eunice Kennedy Shriver National Institute of Child Health and Human Development (NICHD)

"*Sacrifices* explores the unique experiences of African American women and shows how too much sacrifice, often made in the name of family and racial progress, can cause profound harm to our bodies and mind. Writing with empathy, tenderness, and grace—and from a wellspring of personal and professional experience—Dr. Andrea Sullivan serves up a timely road map to true health and wellness. Her advice is practical, no-nonsense, science based, and honest. It will uplift you—and change your life."

—Marilyn Milloy, Former Deputy Editor of *AARP Magazine*

"*The Sacrifices of Superwomen* is a treasure for millions of women in search of healing. Dr. Sullivan speaks in the powerful voice of an author with almost forty years of medical experience. Her compassionate words are as profound as her sage advice, for Andrea Sullivan is a superwoman herself."

—Paul Mittman, ND, EdD, President and CEO of Sonoran University of Health Sciences

"This book is a must-read! Convicting, revealing, instructive, life-changing! Dr. Andrea Sullivan digs deep, peeling back multiple layers of issues that trap so-called superwomen beneath the heavy weights of exhaustion, depression, stress, and disease. Sullivan speaks hard truths about our unhealthy relationships with bad food, bad habits, and ourselves as she declares, 'Enough' with the guilt, anger, resentment, and shame that have caught many of us in a vicious cycle of illness and medication. As a patient and true believer, I feel much better and am convinced that the most direct path from chronic disease to wellness and well-being is exercise, more natural foods, natural remedies, and better sleep! I can now joyfully shed my superwoman cape!"

—Pat Lawson Muse, News Anchor (retired), NBC4-TV, Washington, DC

"I completed Howard University Medical School in 1975, six years before my future friend, Dr. Andrea Sullivan, began school to become a doctor of naturopathic medicine. We were both trained in many of the same courses the first two years, such as anatomy, physiology, microbiology, etc. The last two years, we trained in clinical work, which differed between the practices. As she states in her treatise, allopathic or Western medicine's emphasis was/is how to diagnose and manage a disease most often based on laboratory tests, specialized studies, and physician experience. The emphasis in naturopathic treatment is a holistic approach to care, including history of the patient (often back to childhood), nutrition, and exercise, followed by a plan to improve one's health.

"As for most people, there are things that 'we don't know that we don't know.' Some will never have an 'aha moment,' and it's OK. I have had mine. Hence, Dr. Sullivan and I have consulted and referred patients back and forth for many years. We have trust in the other's abilities, and our goal remains to have optimal health for our patients. This treatise is full of knowledge and wisdom. I highly recommend it for anyone who is serious about getting healthy and/or staying healthy."

—Caryl G. Mussenden, Obstetrician-Gynecologist, MD

"I absolutely love this book. It is a true treasure filled with educational gems and knowledge that continues to guide me and my family throughout life. I've learned to use the gems in this book to teach my children to love themselves in ways that help us unlearn and relearn in the most proper ways to secure a healthy future. Thank you, Dr Sullivan, for this gem of a book!"

—Diamond P., Membership Marketing, Costco

"What Dr Sullivan has written is a lovely, comprehensible, and commonsensical book that I would like to place in the hands of every person I know, every person I encounter on the sidewalk, and especially every twenty-something—including myself twenty-some years ago. Her words integrate different aspects of life that contemporary science likes to tease apart into specifics. And yet that same science continues to show us how integrated everything truly is. More importantly, this is a guidebook by which to understand how to navigate life. Thank you for creating a book in which the thread is honesty and an intention to help. Thank you for these reminders and new awarenesses."

—Renee Schettler, Senior Editor at *Yoga Journal*

"*The Sacrifices of Superwomen* combines all that is needed for women of color to come into balance: the history of present health concerns and how to reclaim self-worth and true well-being. Dr. Sullivan provides a clear, detailed path for a life of vitality. A must-read for all the superwomen out there!"

—Dr. Puja Shah, Award-Winning Author of *For My Sister*

"Dr. Sullivan shares historical information, personal stories, and case studies of women who have focused so much on giving without replenishing themselves. Much is related to some form of discrimination. Over time, this leads to compromised health and well-being. She provides natural remedies to improve health, and practices and affirmations to encourage self-care and self-love. While the examples she provides are mostly centered around Black women, the content and remedies are applicable to all women. This topic also hits close to home because I have studied alternative healing practices and recently wrote my doctoral thesis on boundaries and self-love, so the themes Dr. Sullivan raised were a wonderful reinforcement of many of the lessons I've learned."

—Sonee Singh, DDiv, Multi-Award-Winning Author of *Lonely Dove, Soul-Seeker Poetry Collection*, and *Can You Be*

"I found Dr. Andrea Sullivan after successfully completing treatment for breast cancer. By the time I reached her, I realized I'd been pouring from an empty cup that had dried many years before walking through her office door. Since then, Dr Sullivan has provided so much guidance while walking closely beside me on a journey to wellness. *The Sacrifices of Superwomen* is filled with many of the steps that she has consistently emphasized to me in order to reach true healing from the inside out. It's a book that has helped me refill that empty cup I had when I met Dr. Sullivan. Reading *The Sacrifices of Superwomen* means being able to access her very keen wisdom at your fingertips. It is a must-read for not only those of us who are guilty of putting the needs of others before ourselves but also anyone looking to cultivate a happy, healthy, and whole lifestyle. It is not just a one-time read, either. It is a handbook for life—your best life."

—J. Stewart, Teacher

The Sacrifices of Superwomen: Natural Remedies to Restore Balance
by Andrea D. Sullivan, PhD, ND, DSc h. c.

© Copyright 2023 Andrea D. Sullivan, PhD, ND, DSc h. c.

ISBN 979-8-88824-132-5

All rights reserved. No part of this publication may be reproduced, stored in a retrieval system, or transmitted in any form or by any means—electronic, mechanical, photocopy, recording, or any other—except for brief quotations in printed reviews, without the prior written permission of the author.

Published by

köehlerbooks™

3705 Shore Drive
Virginia Beach, VA 23455
800-435-4811
www.koehlerbooks.com

THE SACRIFICES OF SUPERWOMEN

NATURAL REMEDIES TO RESTORE BALANCE

ANDREA D. SULLIVAN, PHD, ND, DSc h. c.

VIRGINIA BEACH
CAPE CHARLES

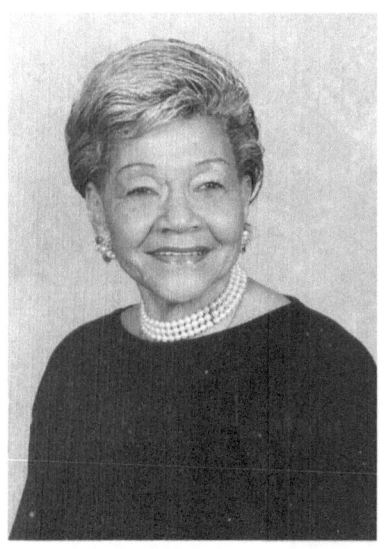

This book is dedicated to the memory
of my mother Mary Lucretia Harris Sullivan
August 22, 1919-September 24, 2019

TABLE OF CONTENTS

Gratitude xv

Introduction: Behind the Cape of a Superwoman xvii

Chapter 1: Consider This 1

Chapter 2: How Did This Happen 8

Chapter 3: The Lives of Superwomen 16

Chapter 4: The Stress of Racism for All of Us 23

Chapter 5: Do Something Different/Take Control 44

Chapter 6: Where Do I Start? Nutrition 65

Chapter 7: Go to Sleep (What a Concept) 91

Chapter 8: Exercise (Baby Steps Are Fine) 100

Chapter 9: Listening to What's Within/
Meditation/Spiritual Exercises 105

Chapter 10: The Truth as I Know It 112

Epilogue 122

Biography 124

Bibliography 126

Endnotes 132

GRATITUDE

Gratitude: The quality of being grateful (warmly or deeply appreciative of kindness or benefits received), or thankful.

Were it not for the grace of Spirit and the never-ending love and support of family (especially Walter and Sean) and friends (Jakki, Ellen, Michael, and Richard), this book would not exist.

Since 1986, I have been blessed to have people come to me and share their stories. They have presented among other diseases, their fears, secrets, shortcomings, deceptions, anger, disappointments, depression, suicidal ideations, and anxiety, with the hope and end goal of healing and wellness. The women who choose me to tell their story honor me. I applaud their tenacity, resilience, and determination to seek something different for themselves and their families. I am humbled by their faith in me and in naturopathic medicine.

It's not easy to bare one's soul. It takes courage. A friend told me once, "It takes great courage to see the face of God." I believe that releasing depression, anxiety, secrets, etc., allows us to see ourselves as we truly are—made in the image of Mother/Father God/All That Is. It takes work, and I am grateful for all of my patients who choose to do the work.

And it took much work to deliver the stories and all the information in this book. For that, I am grateful for Lauren Sheldon of Koehler Books. Her creativity, knowledge, and honest feedback were blessings throughout this process. Dr. Paul Mittman and Suzanne Walker provided much-appreciated detailed editing.

Thank you to Dr. Amy Rothenberg and my agent, Nancy Rosenfeld, for their belief in this project.

I am humbled by the praise given for this book by Donna Brazile, Kim Keenan, Marilyn Milloy, Dr. R. Barbara Gitenstein, Dr. Valerie Maholmes, Dr. Paul Mittman, Pat Lawson Muse, Dr. Caryl Mussenden, D. Patrick, Renee Schettler, Dr. Puja Shah, Dr. Sonee Singh, and J. Stewart. I'm grateful for their willingness to take the time to assist me. Their successes, courage, and passions are examples for me.

Heart and Soul, Andrea D Sullivan, PhD, ND, DHANP, DSc h. c.

INTRODUCTION

Behind the Cape of a Superwoman

Answer honestly.

Are you tired of being overweight or feeling sluggish and unhealthy? Are you tired of the familiar rut of sleeping through your alarm, then finally waking to a diet of coffee and donuts or some other fast-food breakfast sandwich? Are you tired of eating fast food for lunch or, worse, eating no lunch at all? Are you tired of all those muscle aches, joint pain, headaches and backaches? Are you spending too much time on the couch in front of the plug-in drug called TV where you're sitting but not really relaxing? Are you tired of all the medications you have to ingest, some of which are prescribed to lessen the symptoms caused by the medications you have to ingest?

Are you tired of the negative thoughts and feelings—resentment, guilt, fear, and shame–that occupy your brain day in and day out? Are you tired of being irritable, impatient, angry, or anxious? Are you, in the immortal words of iconic Civil Rights activist Fannie Lou Hamer, sick and tired of being sick and tired? And most importantly, are you tired of taking care of everybody but yourself?

I hope you answered yes to all of the above because you cannot continue to do what you have always done—take care of everyone but yourself—and expect a different result. Doing what you've always done and hoping things will change is the definition of insanity. Yet, I understand this brand of insanity. I understand that your heart is big, and you've been conditioned to be a caretaker. I understand you bear others' burdens, even though no one helps you with yours. I understand the responsibility you feel for fulfilling everyone else's needs before you take care of your own. I understand that African American women are the most stressed out and disregarded group in America (with African American men falling in line right behind us). I understand the thrusts and reactions of the Me Too movement, which exploded with the prosecution of Harvey Weinstein and the Black Lives Matter movement, beginning with the acquittal of George Zimmerman in the shooting death of Treyvon Martin, creating more stress for mothers, daughters, sisters, and aunts of young Black men, to the Women's March of 2017, which was spurred by racist, anti-gay, and misogynistic comments made by the former President of the United States, and on to Covid, which exposed the disproportionate deaths of African American women from co-morbidities. We need a new paradigm: to be proactive. We need this book now. If we want to be or support another Michele Obama, Kamala Harris, Ketanji Brown Jackson, or Mellody Hobson, we must be healthy. It is not an option; there are more Amanda Gorman's out there. I understand that African American women overcompensate when we don't feel good about ourselves. And I understand why we have the highest rates of chronic diseases of any group in America.

We are Superwomen.

That origin story is part of a long history. Superwoman was born out of an adaptive response to the abhorrent circumstances of slavery and Jim Crow. Superwoman sacrifices herself for others and succumbs to the "Sojourner Syndrome." Anthropologist Dr. Leith Mullings first advanced the idea of the Sojourner Syndrome in 2002 when she described Sojourner Truth as representative of African American women who resist the "interlocking oppressions of race, class, and gender" that defined their existence for generations. Sojourner sacrificed herself for the good of the collective, took on numerous roles and responsibilities and, as a result, endured an inordinate amount of stress that impacted her health (Mullings, 2002).[1] At age 86, Sojourner died from leg ulcers resulting from untreated diabetes.

Allow me to introduce four modern-day Superwomen: Diane,

Darlene, Mary, and Letitia.

Diane, an African American woman in her late 30s, came to me complaining of constipation, thyroid problems, joint pain, and high blood pressure. She was a pleasant, kind woman who was short in stature and carried more weight than she wanted. She had a muscular body type. Diane was stressed out from raising her grandson, working a demanding federal government job, and dealing with the emotional blow of being passed over for promotion by a young White man whom she had trained.

As I probed a little deeper into Diane's background, she recounted what she termed a "normal" childhood: her father was abusive and an alcoholic, her mother was abused, and her brother, who committed suicide, was verbally abusive. To escape the pain of her upbringing, Diane married young and gave birth to a daughter who became a teenage mother. After marrying, Diane soon discovered her husband was being unfaithful to her. While she was going through the storm of a painful divorce, Diane's father died suddenly from a heart attack. If that wasn't bad enough, Diane's mother blamed her for the anguish and stress her father suffered, and the two of them remained estranged for years.

Darlene was a retired mother and grandmother in her late 60s when she came to see me. She was taking seventeen different medications. She had prescriptions for diabetes, hypertension, and elevated cholesterol levels to name a few. She was of medium height and weight with a sadness that surrounded her as she entered my office. Through tears, she told me about her depression. It began when her husband left her to marry another woman with three children, she told me. She said her husband was mean, violent, and verbally abusive, even after he left. She sought refuge in another relationship, but that soon ended. Darlene had raised her two children and a nephew— the son of her sister who had passed on. Now, just when she felt she should have been sitting back and enjoying her golden years, she became saddled with the burden of raising three of her grandchildren.

Mary, also retired, came to me after being diagnosed with fibromyalgia, high cholesterol, hyperthyroidism, depression, and insomnia. After she went through a nasty divorce and subsequently had to raise her three children alone, Mary never slept well. Mary found out during her divorce proceedings that her husband, a drug addict with erratic behavior, had fathered other children while they were married. While he was not physically abusive to her, she never felt safe with him—or supported.

"My husband was always off chasing other women. So many things were coming at me. I was overwhelmed, anxious, and feeling I had no control. Even now I am doing so much for others and not for myself," she said. "I make sure others are well, but not me. They cannot find out what is really wrong with me. I am raising my six-year-old granddaughter because my daughter is on drugs, and I take care of my 94-year-old mother. There is always so much to do and so little time to do it. I have fears about my health and having enough money. I feel backed into a corner and afraid I cannot get things done. I just feel things are out of control."

Letitia is a pleasant woman who said she thought her immune system was weak because she had so many allergies and headaches. She had a few extra pounds for her height and thought she was obese. Upon being asked about her stress, she said her main stress was from raising her four children as a single mom for many years. However, as she talked further, I realized her stress and subsequent weakened immune system was a result of much more than being a single mom.

She rather casually told me of her history of abuse—physically, mentally/emotionally, and sexually. Her self-esteem was questionable, and she did not speak up for herself as a result. She was angry and didn't express that emotion either. She worked hard and had a good job, yet she was hesitant to advance any further. Letitia's self-esteem disabled her from thinking she could perform the tasks necessary to do the job effectively.

My patients' stories remind me of a time when I was weighed down by my own Superwoman cape. At 26, I earned a PhD in Sociology and Criminology from the University of Pennsylvania. I then taught graduate and undergraduate students at Howard University. When I was 29, I was working as a Special Assistant for Urban Policy for Dr. Patricia Roberts Harris, the first African American woman to be appointed a Presidential cabinet member. My typical workday went non-stop from eight in the morning until six or seven at night. Pretty soon, I was burnt out, and I knew I needed help.

I turned to Dr. James L. D'Adamo desperate to lose the weight, the chronic fatigue, and the terrible acne that had been plaguing me. During my first visit to Dr. D'Adamo, a naturopathic physician, I became aware that much of my "dis-ease" had to do with the experiences with racism I had endured growing up as an African American woman where everything from the bread to the milk to models on TV were white. As we began peeling back the layers of my past, namely sexual molestation by a neighbor across the street, relationships with unfaithful men, and the low self-esteem that followed, I shared with him that despite earning good grades in high school, my guidance counselor told me I should become a domestic worker. I told him about the shame and humiliation I felt upon hearing that and the shame that overwhelmed me when my White high school friends hid me in the basement as soon as their parents' friends came over. I also told him about the shame I felt about being bisexual. Always wanting to compensate for my perceived inadequacies and sense of inferiority, I had worn myself out.

The stress that results from racism, classism, sexism—any "ism" you can name— often promotes low self-esteem, negative thought patterns, and poor nutritional habits, all of which provide a fertile ground for dis-ease to develop. Additionally, African Americans contend with the everyday challenges of racism from without as well as colorism from within. In our own families, many African American women are treated differently based on the lightness or darkness of our skin tone.

African American women also bear the brunt of the effects

of job discrimination, single parenting, and partners and family members suffering from drug and alcohol addictions. Some of us have suffered sexual abuse at the hands of a father, brother, mother, uncle, babysitter, grandfather, or neighbor. These traumas influence how we view the world and ourselves and how we handle life's daily happenings. Years of mental, emotional, and spiritual neglect and abuse negatively affect our physical health and wellbeing.

Then, and only then, do we seek help. Far too many women come to me after they've hit their breaking point—engulfed in their Superwoman capes, addicted to fast food, wobbling on aching joints, and popping more pills than the law should allow.

It is time to declare ENOUGH!

I wrote *The Sacrifices of Superwomen: Natural Remedies to Restore Balance* because I want African American women to stop dying faster and younger than White women. I want women of color to stop dying from cancer at higher rates. I want African American women to eat less fried chicken, drink more water, go to sleep before midnight, and exercise for at least ten minutes a day three times a week. I want us to stand up and have the courage to say "No!" I want us to forgive ourselves and stop judging ourselves and others. I want every woman to know who she is spiritually and to recognize she is a precious soul where God resides. If we are truly committed to beginning the healing process, we have to develop new habits, rehearse new thought patterns, and make different choices. How do we get there? We have to start with a new understanding about the value of our health.

The Sacrifices of Superwomen: Natural Remedies to Restore Balance was created to save lives, decrease morbidity, and alleviate and heal dis-ease in African American women. This book will inspire you to take control of your emotional, physical, and spiritual health and wellbeing. Instead of spending your money on the best clothes, cars, jewels, and handbags, this book will show you how to invest in your health and create the kind of wealth money can't buy. This book offers a practical toolkit that helps you make yourself a priority, repair your body and, most importantly, prevent its breakdown.

The Sacrifices of Superwomen: Natural Remedies to Restore Balance will show you how to begin the practice of caring for and loving yourself. Even if you choose to continue to be a Superwoman who guides, protects, supports, nourishes, nurtures, and loves others, you can also choose to love and nourish yourself. *Giving from a place of lack just won't work.* We must learn to give from our own well of abundance, strength, and sustenance. It's time to don a cape woven with threads of awareness and wisdom on how to cultivate robust health and well-being. Let me ask you: do you honestly think God put you here to be sick, stressed out, and forever on the verge of a breakdown? The opposite is true. You are entitled to have good health and have it more abundantly.

This isn't your typical, quick fix, Hollywood fad-diet book. It is a journey of discovery into the world of naturopathic medicine and your own power to heal. Naturopathic medicine may sound foreign to women of color, but it has been the key to saving my patients' lives. Indeed, naturopathic medicine has been saving lives for centuries. *Naturopaths are medical professionals who treat people, not conditions. Naturopaths carefully consider a patient's physical, emotional, mental, and spiritual states of being since each serves as the root of both dis-ease and the healing of dis-ease. Naturopaths work with patients to remedy the causes, not just the outward signs of their illnesses. In doing so, naturopaths prescribe natural substances and lifestyle changes to aid in healing and overall robust health.* I tell my patients, "Doctor means teacher, not God. We will work together as a team. You cannot drop your body off and pick it up at five o'clock like a car. You have to get involved."

The Sacrifices of Superwomen: Natural Remedies to Restore Balance is about using your strengths and discipline to heal and save yourself. And save yourself you must. You cannot afford to do nothing in hopes that the systems which have been oppressing you for centuries will somehow rally to save you. And not just the socio/economic and political systems in America fraught with racism, sexism, and discriminatory practices. Also, the sick care system. In 1966, while in Chicago to make a presentation to the Medical Committee for Human Rights, Dr. Martin Luther King, Jr. said this to the reporters: "Of all the forms of inequality, injustice in healthcare is the most shocking and inhuman." Of course, the history of this inhumane care goes back to slavery when it was a common thought among slave owners that slaves had different diseases than whites. It was also a common thought that slaves tolerated more pain than whites (a theory still percolating in some medical environments; hence, we are under-treated with pain medication). There was much experimentation—amputations, caesarians—performed on African slaves to prove that we could tolerate more pain than Whites. Now we hardly get preventive services, wait longer for sick care services, and may receive fewer or none at all in many places in the country. Covid-19 was an example of the latter, as people of color were turned away from hospitals even though they couldn't breathe and had oxygen levels below 80.[2] And the lack of testing sites in underserved areas were an additional problem.[3] This system has for too long been one of discrimination, bringing more pain and suffering at times than the diagnoses.

The book is designed to help you discover how to restore overall balance and wellbeing to your mind and body. Throughout *The Sacrifices of Superwomen*, you will discover specific life-saving changes that can help you manage and combat the negative effects of stress, the Sojourner Syndrome, and the Superwoman persona. Yes! We can retreat from the brink of disaster by reclaiming naturopathic medicine. I write reclaiming since our African ancestors practiced that encompassing form of medicine even though they didn't call it naturopathy.

Reading *The Sacrifices of Superwomen: Natural Remedies to*

Restore Balance will assist you along your path to robust health and wellness by suggesting necessary lifestyle changes. On the pages that follow, I will teach you about proper nutrition and personal growth and the stress-reduction techniques that changed my life and the lives of many others. I will also address the unique experiences in African American communities that have given rise to behavioral adaptations that negatively impact our health. This book will not right all social wrongs or miraculously reverse all dis-ease. It will not end racism and discrimination in health care.

My hope is it will empower you and provide a foundation to embark on a journey toward wellness. You can do this. Think about it: African Americans survived the Middle Passage, slavery, the Black Codes, Jim Crow segregation, the war on drugs, and today we're battling the New Jim Crow. If we can survive those oppressions, surely we can change our negative thinking and our less-than-optimal eating habits.

The truth is, we can do anything. Many have led the way: Harriet Tubman, Fannie Lou Hammer, Dr. Anna Julia Cooper, Rosa Parks, Coretta Scott King, and Betty Shabazz. So if you're still thinking you're too busy saving everyone else to devote time and attention to your own physical, emotional, and spiritual needs, then how about this: if you won't do it for yourself, then do it for your great grandmother, your grandmother, your children, or grandchildren. Better yet, JUST DO IT—for you.

It's time to say enough! Enough of the sedentary lifestyle, watching TV, and snacking. Enough of eating poorly and being in a state of chronic fatigue. Enough struggling with your weight and Enough putting off exercising regularly. Enough of the gossip, negative self-talk, not loving yourself, and not recognizing that you are your greatest asset. Enough of saying "Yes" all the time and doing for everyone except yourself. Enough with thinking it is better to give than to receive since giving and receiving are part of the same cycle of abundance. Stop dimming your light so others can shine.

Stop denying your worthiness. Stop the guilt, anger, resentment, and shame you carry. Let's reduce the dis-eases, and medications. Let's RESTORE BALANCE!

SACRIFICE

The offering of animal, plant or human life or of some object to a deity, as in propitiation of homage; the person, animal. or thing so offered; the surrender or destruction of something valued for the sake of something having a higher or more pressing claim; something so surrendered or lost.

    Synonyms—loss, deprivation, privation, forfeit, expense, cost, damage, destruction, ruin... .

CHAPTER 1

Consider This

Black women will do anything for people they love, but not for themselves. "Some other time" never comes.

—Darlene

The Hard, Cold Facts – The Results of Being a Superwoman

For too long I have heard many of my patients echo Darlene—almost verbatim. What they are admitting to is that they sacrifice themselves daily. They're stating that the needs and desires of everyone in their inner circle come before their own. Every day, Black women attempt to give of themselves, not from an overflow but from lack—a lack of time, energy, or money. The consequences of this are not pretty.

Look at these statistics:

- 56.7 percent of African American women over the age of 20 have hypertension as compared to only 36.7 percent of white women and 36.8 percent of Hispanic women in the same age bracket. (Ostchega Y, 2020)[4]
- While more white women are likely to have breast cancer, we have a higher mortality rate—an average of five African American women die from breast cancer every day. (Richardson, Henley, Miller, Massetti, & Thomas, 2016)[5]

- Four out of five African American women are overweight or obese.
- African American women die at a 50 percent higher death rate from diabetes than White women, (Diabetes and African Americans, 2021)[6]
- African American women have higher rates of HPV, human papillomavirus, and cervical cancer, with mortality rates double those of White women (Banister CE, 2015)[7]
- Only 35 percent of African American lesbian and bisexual women have had a mammogram in the past two years, compared to 60 percent of white lesbian and bisexual women. (Kimball, 2020)[8]
- African American women have greater mortality than Caucasian women from CAD (coronary artery disease), hypertension, stroke, and CHF. (Congestive Heart Failure) The mortality rate from CAD is 69 percent higher in Black women than in White women. Mortality for Black females from hypertension is 352 percent higher than for White females.[9] Age-adjusted stroke death rates are 54 percent higher in African American than in Caucasian women. Incidence, prevalence, and morbidity figures for CAD, hypertension, stroke, and CHF are all higher for African American females than for Caucasian females. (Williams, 2009)[10]

The COVID-19 crisis has shone a spotlight on the health disparities that have existed in African Americans communities for centuries. African Americans are disproportionately represented in the cases of and deaths from COVID-19. In states where Black communities make up a small portion of the population, nearly half of all deaths are members of that community. And in larger cities like Chicago where the population is 30 percent Black, we are half of the cases and 70 percent of those who died. In Louisiana, 70 percent of those who died are Black, while making up only one-third of the population.[11] Having asthma increases one's risk of getting COVID-19 and related complications. African Americans were already three times more likely to die from asthma related causes. African American women were 20 percent more likely to have asthma in 2015 (US Department of Health and Human Services, Office of minority Health), because 75 percent of the black population live in areas that border a factory or refinery (Clean Air task Force Report, NAACP 2017). According to the Asthma and Allergy Foundation of America, African American women have the highest rates of death due to asthma.

These circumstances are directly related in part to African American women being in service positions that do not allow for teleworking (we make up 30 percent of the workforce that are caregivers outside the home), utilizing public transportation, living in poor housing and neighborhoods with toxicity in the air and water, no access to quality health care, and of course the aforementioned pre-existing health issues. And though taking care of our immune systems is more important now than ever before, the economic conditions in African American communities function to worsen our health challenges:

- US Bureau of Labor Statistics reported the unemployment rate for African American women over 20 years of age is twice that of White men and since December 2020 our unemployment rate is 8.4 percent compared to White women, at 5.7 percent. The number of White women in the labor force grew by 263,000 in December, but the number of Black women fell by 153,000, and we are paid 62 cents on the dollar. White women are paid 79 cents on the dollar. (Corbett, 2020) (Survey, 2022)[12,13]
- The poverty rate for all African Americans in the District of Columbia in 2018 was 27 percent.
- African American families with children under the age of 18

headed by a single mother have the highest rate of poverty at 46 percent (nationwide) as compared to only 8.4 percent of families headed by married African American couples.
- Thirty percent of African American women work in service positions compared to 17 percent of White women. Black women's labor market history reveals deep-seated race and gender discrimination. (n.d., retrieved from https://www.epi.org/blog/black-womens-labor-market-history-reveals-deep-seated-race-and-gender-discrimination/) And almost 19 percent of African American women lost their jobs between February and April 2020 at the onset of the pandemic. Now 80 percent of us are primary bread winners and are heads of household.
- African American women experience poverty at higher rates than African American men and women from all other ethnic groups except Native American women; a quarter of Black women in the US live in poverty. Black women are 3.6 times more likely than White women to be single heads of households with children under the age of 18. (Bieiweis, 2020)[14]

The societal challenges enumerated above keep African American women locked in a vicious cycle. When a single mother is struggling with poverty, she may not have the time or money to plan wholesome meals for her family. Easy accessibility to refined, high-fat food makes quick on-the-go meals the solution to feeding her family. Exercise may not even be a consideration with her full schedule.

Thus, too many women are following in the footsteps of Sojourner, someone who can seemingly do it all but sacrifices herself for the collective good. Sojourner's resiliency and strength in the face of the most inhumane circumstances were heroic, and she deserves praise. But when an entire nation of women tries to take on that burden, giving more than we have and running up a debt on our emotional, physical, and spiritual resources, we pay a terrible price.

Is It Really "Soul" Food?

As a society, Americans do not value health nor recognize the impact poor health has on their lives. What else would we expect after being at the mercy of a society and a culture that promotes eating chemically-laden substances and calling it food? For so long, Americans have been fooled into thinking that just because it tastes good, it's good for you. Many have been indulging in the opposite of what Random House dictionary defines as food, which is "any nourishing substance, eaten, drunk, or otherwise taken into the body to sustain life, provide energy, and promote growth." That definition certainly doesn't sound like the Standard American Diet (SAD).

And while it has become trendy to "eat well" or "buy organic," eating better isn't pocket-friendly for many Americans. The average consumer has to pay more for food that is free of chemicals and pesticides, and actually good for you. Despite this new awareness of clean eating and eco-friendly, organic cooking, many African Americans are still indulging in diets that we affectionately call "soul food." Soul food has its origins in slavery when enslaved people were given scraps from their enslavers' tables, scraps including pork, dark meat chicken, and saturated oils, that today lead to multiple illnesses. It's soul food, alright. This food may provide warm feelings and memories of home, but it may take you to your home-going service faster than you anticipated.

Are We Sacrificing Good Looks for Well-Being?

Health has not traditionally been a top priority for African American women. There are many reasons for this: distrust of medical doctors, lack of financial resources and sick care delivery systems, putting ourselves last, and not making healthcare a priority. However, we live in communities where our fuller bosoms and curvier hips are celebrated. White Americans and African Americans have almost opposite perspectives about what is acceptable regarding weight.

Anorexia and bulimia continue to be huge problems, particularly for White female teens, while in African American culture it is acceptable to be heavier and endowed with larger buttocks.

Historically and currently in South Africa, having more weight has been viewed as something positive. There is a dignity and respect associated with weight that represents good health and a good life. Maasai men in central Africa have "fattening periods" to be more attractive to the women. It is thought that heavier bodies protect against wasting and illness. In many African cultures today, when a person is thin, it is assumed they are going through a difficult time, a severe illness, drug addiction, or even battling HIV.

While our African brothers and sisters have packed on the pounds with traditional yams, cassava plants, and rice, we in America think we can do the same with yams that are smothered with marshmallows or greens that have been cooked beyond their nutritional value or soaked with ham hocks and turkey necks. While most of our African counterparts are walking for miles each day,[15] the most exercise many African Americans get is walking from the front door to our cars. Our curves are indeed beautiful, but we can't sacrifice our wellbeing for shapely curves.

Choosing Style Over Health

Our perceived lack of purposeful contributions, whether from evaluations from our bosses or partners, unfulfilled relationships and dreams, the need for instant gratification, or of advertisers encouraging food addictions, keep us romanticizing desired clothing, shoes, and material things more than good health.

A potential patient told me that she could not afford to eat well, but she regularly spends upwards of $300 per month to color her hair and maintain her weave. Her monthly "looking good" budget also includes funds for pedicures and manicures, shopping sprees at Nordstrom, and weekly gambling at the local casino. Several of my patients have canceled appointments with me, they said, because they'd spent too much money on Amazon.

I'm not here to judge anyone's choices. We all have different priorities when it comes to evaluating what's most important in our lives. *The Sacrifices of Superwomen: Natural Remedies to Restore Balance* is here to be your resource and your toolkit for creating change. New habits, new thought patterns, and new choices must be made in order to heal your wounds and move forward. I am not naive. I know that changing your eating habits, exercising, drinking water, meditating, sleeping better, and thinking positive thoughts will not take care of all the ills we suffer, as we still must contend with an unequal and discriminatory sick care system. I do know that if you have the intention to do any one of those things mentioned above, the methods will show up and you may be able to avoid premature involvement in that system.

Begin this journey by starting from where you are—right now. Accept the past and be grateful for today. From this place of acceptance and gratitude, I will show you how to take baby steps toward life-saving changes so that you're LIVING a life toward wellness EVERY DAY.

Say this out loud:

I AM LOVED. I AM WELL. I AM GOD'S CHILD.

CHAPTER 2

How Did This Happen?

Not asking for help is an issue. I could appear vulnerable. Being hurt is the fear... even playing Superwoman, you get hurt.

—Diane

Sojourner Truth – Sista Warrior

Sojourner Truth, whose given name was Isabella Baumfree, was born enslaved in New York State around 1787. After her father was captured in Ghana, West Africa and her mother in Guinea, they were both sold into slavery. Sojourner was separated from her family at a young age and raised under oppressive conditions. She witnessed the sale of her brothers and sisters and later her son. Sojourner was no stranger to heartache.

She was sold for the first time at age nine for 100 dollars and a flock of sheep after her enslaver died. Sojourner labored for three other enslavers and was often abused physically, sexually, and of course emotionally. She had three other enslavers after that, and she continued to be physically, emotionally, and sexually abused. She was ultimately forced to marry an enslaved man whom she did not love. She gave birth to a son James, who died in childhood, another son Peter, and three daughters—Sophia, Elizabeth, and Diana. Diana was conceived when Sojourner was raped by one of her enslavers.

Sojourner ran away in 1827, the year before New York's law abolishing slavery took effect. Taking only her infant daughter

Sophia, she escaped to a nearby abolitionist family. That family paid 20 dollars to secure her freedom and later helped her win a lawsuit seeking the return of her five-year-old son Peter, who had been illegally sold into slavery in Alabama. (Michals, 2015)[16] After Peter's disappearance from the ship where he worked, Sojourner felt she was called by God to travel or "sojourn" and speak the truth. Consequently, she changed her name to Sojourner Truth and became an abolitionist speaker.

While on one abolitionist tour, Sojourner attended the Ohio Women's Rights convention. Her famous spontaneous speech at the convention in 1851, "Ain't I a Woman," spoke to the oppression and resilience of African American women and the contrasting deferential treatment accorded to wealthy White women. (Craig, 2002)[17]

Women were perceived as the "weaker sex," and wealthy aristocratic White women were to focus solely on household duties and child rearing and leave field labor to enslaved Black women. Thus, Black women suffered under the weight of racism and sexism. Enslaved Black women suffered economic exploitation, family dissolution, sexual exploitation, and of course forced childbearing to produce a labor pool for their enslavers. Additionally, enslaved women were used as subjects in medical experiments. (Winkler)[18]

Sexism, The Sojourner Syndrome and Superwoman

In the mid 1700's, American colonies based their law on English common law, which made the husband and wife essentially one person legally. The oppression from sexism was the focus of The Declaration of Sentiments of 1848, as it was called, at the first woman's rights convention in Seneca Falls, NY. Attended by 68 women and 32 men, including Fredrick Douglass, the Declaration of Sentiments underscored the following concerns: married White women were legally without rights; they could not sue or be sued; women could not vote until 1920; married White women had no property rights;

husbands had legal power over their wives and could do things like beat or imprison them with impunity; women could not enter into contracts; divorce and child custody favored men; women did not have legal rights to their children; women could not work outside the home;[19] women were essentially servants to their husbands; colleges and universities would not accept women; and most occupations were closed to women, especially medicine and law. (Knisely, 2017)[20]

Further attempts to suppress women can be seen in examples of Supreme Court cases. The Supreme Court in Bradwell v. Illinois, 83 US 130 (1872) ruled that a state had the right to exclude a married woman from practicing law. In 1869, the territory of Wyoming passed America's first law allowing women to vote. However, in Minor v. Happersett, 88 US 162 (1875), the Court declared that a state could prohibit a woman from voting. The court said women constituted a special category of nonvoting citizens.

Women could not serve on juries until 1960, and could not work while pregnant until 1970. In the late 1800s, passports were beginning to be standardized. At that time a single woman could be issued a passport in her own name, but a married woman was listed as an anonymous add-on to her husband's document. Interestingly, the US passport includes 143 inspirational quotes from notable Americans, and only one belongs to a woman—African American scholar, educator, and activist, Anna J Cooper. In 1892 she wrote, "The cause of freedom is not the cause of a race or a sect, a party or a class—it is the cause of humankind, the very birthright of humanity." (Cooper, 1892)[21]

The current lack of autonomy and respect for women is seen in the Supreme Court's overturning of Roe v. Wade, which said the Constitution conferred the right of women to have an abortion. After 50 years of it being held as law, all states are now able to make abortion illegal even in the case of rape or incest. Given that African American women have higher mortality rates in childbearing, what else may be the outcome of this ruling? In the case of incest, there could be genetic problems, congenital disabilities, and premature births, to mention only a few physical concerns. The spiritual, mental, emotional, physical, and financial ramifications are endless and even more traumatic if the circumstance of the birth is due to rape.

Today, women continue to be treated unequally worldwide compared to our male counterparts. The Oxfam Organization tells us that, on average, women are paid 24 percent less than men for comparable work, across all regions and sectors. And nearly two-thirds of the world's illiterate adults are women. Here at home in the US, the literacy rate for females above 15 years of age is less than 83 percent, while for males the literacy rate is 90 percent. This impacts greatly on one's ability to secure and maintain employment. Historically, it was decided women were better suited for housework and childcare, so a formal education was not important. Some of my older patients have told me that their fathers did not support them to go to college as they did their brothers and in fact dissuaded them from attending any institution of higher learning.

Combine this history with the experience of slavery for the African woman in North America and you get the Sojourner Syndrome—a symbolic representation that traces our current health disparities to the roles, responsibilities, and inequitable circumstances that have plagued African American women for centuries.

During slavery there was little external motivation to do or be anything except a slave (other than freedom, of course). The fact that many enslaved people were not allowed to marry someone of their choice (as in the case of Sojourner) often led to a lack of responsibility and accountability within our communities. Even if they wanted to be the head of the household, enslaved African men had limited opportunities to do so. In his book, *Slavery* (1971), Stanley M. Elkins states "'Sambo', the typical plantation slave was docile but irresponsible, loyal but lazy, humble but chronically given to lying and stealing; his behavior was full of infantile silliness and his talk inflated with childish exaggeration. His relationship with his master was one of utter dependence and childlike attachment." Elkins asks the question, "Was Sambo real?" Clearly even in the 1900s, and maybe today, this character was seen as the product of racial inheritance. And with these circumstances came the lack of a two-person household structure and the integrity of a family unit for enslaved Africans. If you were married, there was the constant threat the marriage would end with the nod of the master. Life was chaotic and unstable. Enslaved African women, if they were allowed to keep their offspring, had to be responsible for the family.

Now more and more African American women are heads of households. African American women either can't find a job or work several jobs while bearing the responsibility for the economic, social, psychological, moral, cultural, and spiritual responsibilities of our families and communities. Yet within the immediate community, there's a lack of positive role models, including models for intimacy, love, and conflict resolution. African American women are under consistent and persistent psychological, emotional, social, and physical stress that greatly contributes to their health disparities.

Years after being denigrated as chattel slaves, African American women were depicted negatively in popular culture as "Mammy" or "Aunt Jemima." This characterization served to keep African American women inept, less than ignorant, and devoted to the White family. Then of course there was the "Jezebel" persona, which arose from African American women being blamed for being sexually exploited during slavery. In response to these characterizations, the reference to African American women as "Superwoman" was born to highlight the positive attributes that developed as a result of oppression and adversity. (Woods-Giscombé, 2010)[22]

The dehumanizing experiences we've endured for generations created a legacy of independence, strength, and self-determination. Our resilience and perseverance enabled us to survive socially and economically. We have learned how to protect ourselves, our families, and our communities. These adaptations have led us to become

Superwomen. But being a Superwoman comes at great cost. African American women who have been vigilant, strong, resilient, and brave in the face of tragedy have also suffered from disproportionate health disparities and a shortened life expectancy. Even Superman had his kryptonite.

In sociology the result of this adaptation is called "weathering," a term coined by Dr. Arline Geronimus in 1992 at the University of Michigan. (Geronimus, 1992)[23] Random House Dictionary defines weathering as "the process by which natural agents, as wind and water, act upon exposed rock, causing it to disintegrate to sand and soil; wear away or change the appearance or texture of something by long exposure to the air; withstand difficulty or danger; the process of wearing or being worn by long exposure to the atmosphere." In this case the "atmosphere," "the wind, water, and natural agents," though not limited to the following, is one of marginalization, social, health and racial injustice, the delayed response to the winds and water of Katrina or the Flint Michigan water crisis, and generational economic disparities, growing worse due to Covid- 19. And then there are the jobs that cannot be remote or the lack of internet access for learning for many African American children.

In my first book, *A Path to Healing: A Guide to Wellness for Body, Mind, and Soul,* I made it clear that I believe racism is the greatest dis-ease in America; a destructive and violent source of sickness, with far reaching tentacles. Due to racism and our sick care system, we have been the exposed rock, disintegrating into sand and soil.

It is no secret African American women are disproportionately represented in every major chronic disease category. African American women have greater morbidity and mortality rates than White women for nearly every major illness. (Howell, 2018)[24] According to the Centers for Disease Control and Prevention, 38.1 percent of all African American men over the age of 20 are obese, and 37.6 percent of the same population are hypertensive. For women it is worse: 54.2 percent of all African American women over age 20 are obese, 80 percent are overweight, and 45.7 percent are hypertensive (as compared to 28 percent of White women in the same category). (Obesity and African Americans, 2019)[25]

It's time to invest in lifestyle changes that decrease morbidity and disease. It's true, many women do not know what to do to create healthy habits. Others do know, yet they continue to make poor choices. Instead of spending money on things that support us in leading healthier balanced lives, some of us buy the best clothing, cars, jewelry, nails, hair, handbags, and tattoos. Retail therapy is not, in and of itself, bad, but if you don't prioritize your health, all you're left with are some very expensive handbags to go along with your hypertension.

I grew up at a time when there was talk of revolution. Though what was being said about racism and discrimination was true, I was not willing to hurt anyone because of the color of their skin or opposing beliefs. For me, violence was never an option. Now we commit acts of violence toward ourselves and each other regularly. With every indiscretion in thought, word, or deed, with every poor dietary choice, we are slowly but surely shortening our time on this planet and inviting suffering. It's time to begin the health and wellness revolution. We must be revolutionary in our thinking, speaking, vision, and behavior. We must empower ourselves. We must take care of ourselves by creating healthier lifestyles for our minds, bodies, and souls. The evolution/revolution must begin within each of us, and it must begin now.

We will not achieve healing by blaming and despising others for their actions; we will achieve it by empowering ourselves. When we heal ourselves, we help to heal our neighbors, and when we heal our neighbors, we help to heal the ailing body of humankind. Each of us can take responsibility for our own wellness not only through nutrition, stress reduction, and natural therapies, but also by thinking healthier thoughts, speaking kinder words, and participating in greater acts of service.

Let's begin to love more, starting with ourselves. Let's forgive ourselves for judging ourselves and others as wrong. Let's stop the gossip and negative comments about one another and ourselves. Let's stop the thoughts that we are not good enough or smart enough. Let's be aware we have a birthright to have joy and have it more abundantly. Let's commit to a healthy life full of grace. Let's focus on that for which we are grateful and not on what we do not have. Let's respect ourselves and others. Let's respond to life with integrity. Let's break old habits and create new ones.

Only when we sincerely take care of ourselves and become content with who we are can we create peace in ourselves and congeniality with others. By doing so we maintain our health and integrity and put ourselves in a better position to take care of others without expecting anything in return. In my experience, independence and willingness to stand up for ourselves encourages others to do the same. We need a variety of changes to our behavior to reduce stress and begin a private revolution. To change what you receive, you must change who you are. Small things done consistently over time create major changes.

The key to any healing is self-love, which begins with wanting what is better, for us, not for anyone else. We must commit ourselves to long term change, healing and continued self-love. This commitment doesn't end, it is ongoing. With every obstacle, there must be a re-commitment to yourself to focus on the next goal, not the obstacles This book will assist you in creating those commitments and changes. The information in this book will lift you up and fortify you so that the wellness you seek will enable you to respond to life with greater purpose and intention.

Below are the revolutionary words that will propel us forward.

Ready? State boldly:

I AM LOVED. I AM WELL. I AM GOD'S CHILD.

CHAPTER 3

The Lives of Superwomen

I have to get rid of this Superwoman complex.

—Diane

I spent all my life trying to do for others.

—Darlene

We Black women think we can fix everythin.g

—Mary

I have to keep everything balanced and make sure nothing slips through the cracks; I'm trying to stay afloat.

—Letitia

Can naturopathic methods be the key to restoring your well-being and peace of mind? Let's take a closer look at how Diane, Darlene, and Mary took on their health and ultimately took back their lives.

Diane: The Moody / Loner Superwoman

Diane is a 30-something divorced mother and grandmother, whose grandson lives with her and is not kind to her. She tells me she has high blood pressure and thyroid problems. A loner who is easily offended, she is moody and broods a lot when she is stressed out.

Although she doesn't have many friends, she is loyal, responsible, and dependable. However, because of her past experiences, she fears relying on someone and being totally committed. After one of our sessions, she realized how her stress and health problems stemmed from being generous to everyone but herself. She said, "I don't give myself the freedom to do what I should do for myself. I wait to see what everyone else is doing and then I do for myself. I am held back and want to take flight. I have to get rid of this Superwoman complex."

After discussing her symptoms and background, I gave Diane a homeopathic remedy, Natrum muriaticum, which can help patients suffering from moodiness, irritability, and feelings of isolation. I also advised her to record her eating and sleeping patterns and symptoms. During the next visit, Diane commented that she felt less moody and more energetic, and she wasn't as easily offended. After recording her diet, sleep patterns, and mood for five days, she began a detoxification diet and received colon hydrotherapy. The detoxification diet excluded processed foods, white sugar, rice, and bread, and included whole grains and fresh vegetables. She ate fish twice but no red meat. She began exercising regularly and practicing yoga.

By using naturopathic medicine, I was able to treat Diane as a whole person. Naturopathic practitioners treat the underlying causes of illness, not just the symptoms. A conventional, or allopathic doctor, likely would have prescribed a combination of thyroid, blood pressure, and joint pain medications for Diane. A naturopathic approach, using homeopathic medicine and herbal supplements (e.g., I used a combination of garlic, and cordyceps for her blood pressure), helped Diane's body heal itself by removing the barriers to good health. Ultimately, Diane learned how to better respond to familial and work stress, and she changed her poor diet and sleep habits. She and I worked together for two years, and she counted me as one of her primary-care physicians. Once Diane was feeling better and had lowered her blood pressure, she began making better decisions on her own.

Darlene: The Depressed/ Exhausted Superwoman

Darlene, a 50-something early retiree, came to me with headaches, insomnia, depression and diabetes, a condition that afflicted many of her family members. Like many of my patients, she thought getting diabetes was inevitable so she ate lots of sweets, pastries, and candy and, ultimately, fulfilled her own prophecy. Darlene was a caretaker for her father as he recovered from a stroke. She also served as a caretaker for her brother. When they both passed on, she began to take care of her mother who called on her throughout the night. Darlene turned to her comfort foods while she served as caretaker and when immediate family members passed on.

Darlene was irritable and impatient, and spent most of her time alone. She was so exhausted that she fell asleep at work. Ultimately, she had to quit working when her mother's caretakers didn't work out. Darlene felt as though her mother thought more of Darlene's siblings, who were not involved in their mother's care and did not visit her. These same siblings criticized Darlene by saying she wasn't properly caring for their mother. "I thought I was doing good, and they were saying I wasn't," Darlene told me, as she wept. "I feel guilty thinking, 'Did I do enough to help?' I just miss my father, my mother, and my family so much. It is like a hole in my heart. It is torn. I spent all my life trying to do for others, even if they didn't ask me to. I always think I will be fine. I am finding out I am not."

I helped Darlene see the connection between her diet (white flour, white sugar, white rice and canned, processed foods), diabetes, depression, and feelings of inadequacy, and her loss of control. We worked together to build a nutrition plan to help manage her diabetes and found ways for her to access support without looking for comfort food or validation from her siblings. I gave Darlene Salacia oblonga root, a traditional Ayurveda diabetes treatment that stabilizes blood sugar levels and improves kidney function. I also prescribed the herb berberine, which serves the same purpose. I incorporated red sage root, a traditional Chinese medicine for improving circulation; quercetin, an anti-inflammatory nutraceutical; and Ignatia amara, a homeopathic remedy that treats depression and shock from loss of loved ones. After several weeks of treatment, Darlene reported feeling less depressed. After several months of treatment, she had more stable blood sugar levels.

Mary: The Anxious/ Retired Superwoman

Mary, my 70-year-old patient, came to me after being diagnosed with fibromyalgia, high cholesterol, hyperthyroidism, hypertension, depression, and insomnia. Ever since her divorce and her subsequently having to raise her three children alone, Mary hadn't slept well. She seemed anxious. Mary found out during her divorce proceedings that her husband, who was a drug addict with erratic behavior, had fathered children with other women. While he was not physically abusive, she never felt safe or supported by him.

"My husband was always off chasing other women. So many things were coming at me. I was overwhelmed, anxious, and feeling I had no control. Even now I am doing so much for others and not for myself," she said. "I make sure others are well but not me. They cannot find out what is wrong with me. I am raising my six-year-old granddaughter because my daughter is on drugs, and I take care of my 94-year-old mother. There is always so much to do and so little time to do it. I have fears about my health and having enough money. I feel backed into a corner and afraid I cannot get things done. I just feel things are out of control." Mary reasoned that she had failed as a mother because of her daughter's poor choices.

I treated Mary with the homeopathic remedy Argentum nitricum to decrease her anxiety, insomnia, and the sensation of being out of control. Argentum nitricum is given to people who experience the sensation of overwhelm, a pending failure, or the feeling that a catastrophe is about to strike. For Mary, these feelings began in childhood in response to the chaos brought into her home by her alcoholic father. I also prescribed the herbs turmeric and garlic, as well as flax oil, and a combination of zinc, Vitamin C, riboflavin (a B2 vitamin), amino acids, and selenium. These became a part of her daily regimen along with dietary changes.

Letitia: The Allergic/Overweight Superwoman

Letitia came to me in her mid-40s complaining of allergies, headaches, and obesity. The allergies were to cats and dogs and some foods as well, especially raw vegetables. She also had uterine fibroids and, at 5'5", she weighed 245 pounds. She had a problem with concentration and seemed anxious. She said she had been a single parent of four children, always had two to three jobs at the same time, and always had to juggle so many things to make sure her children were prepared. She told me that her mind was constantly racing, keeping everything in balance. She wanted to make sure her health did not deteriorate, and saw her anxiety as a failure. She wanted to be more organized with all she had to do, but was not settled, feeling lost at times and easily distracted. She was very personable and pleasant.

Letitia told me that, during her childhood, her dad was unfaithful to her mother. He would pick Letitia up and, on the way to wherever they were going, he would stop at a women's house. Even before her birth her dad brought his other daughter, who was born while he was married to Letitia's mother, to come live with him and my patient's mother. Her parents argued and occasionally fought. Once her mom had a kettle on the stove and she hit her father over the head with it. Letitia was embarrassed when her friends asked what happened to him.

Also during her childhood, Letitia was sexually abused on several occasions—once by a relative and another time by a stranger. Fortunately, a neighbor saw her being pulled by the man and came into the building where they were. The man ran away. As many women do in these situations, she thought it was her fault. She thought she had done something to provoke and entice this man, this stranger.

At the age of 15, Letitia became pregnant and her father put her out of the house. She went to her aunt's house and subsequently to the mother of her half-sister, eventually living on the street. The brother of her son's father would not let her stay at his home. Ultimately, her son's father was physically abusive and she left him.

The father of her other children was also abusive verbally and physically. This time she was too afraid to leave. She had fears of being hurt and of hurting him. She had thoughts of scalding him with water. After much fighting, trauma, and stress, she was able to leave and find another place to live for herself and her children.

In each of her relationships, the man forced himself on Letitia at one time or another. She had been physically abused in other situations as well and the culmination of these experiences led her to believe she was not worthy, that she was powerless and voiceless. Letitia found herself not speaking up for herself and allowing others to be unkind to her. She lost a job due to discrimination during this time, as well, and managed to again work multiple jobs after finding a replacement. She had suppressed her anger and rather than address the person with whom she was angry, she suffered from road rage and numerous diseases.

Because of her combined history of abuse—mentally/emotionally, physically and sexually—as well as her suppressed anger, low self-esteem, and feelings of unworthiness, I gave her the remedy Staphysagria. I also asked her to record her diet diary for five days and return in a week. I also gave her an herbal tincture (a liquid preparation) of *Ligusticum porteri* (Osha root), *Euphrasia* (Eyebright), *Mahonia aquifolium* (Oregon Grape), and *Armoracia rusticana* (Horseradish) for her allergies and 1.000 mg of Vitamin C twice a day.

As I reflect on the diseases that plague women like Diane, Darlene, Mary, and Letitia, I am acutely aware that these are not exotic, rare, mysterious ailments without treatment or understanding. These conditions are understandable, preventable, and treatable. These women were able to revamp their lives with lifestyle changes and treatments that didn't include pharmaceutical drugs.

During the past 35 years, I have been blessed to be the vessel used to treat or prevent numerous dis-eases and conditions in many people. I love what I do and I am grateful to do it. Naturopathic medicine is constantly evolving and growing, because there is so much available in nature to be used for healing. There is so much research yet to be done.

Naturopathic treatment involves the use of nature and its elements to support the immune system's natural ability to heal. The treatment may include botanical or herbal medicine, nutritional or dietary changes, nutraceuticals (vitamins, minerals, probiotics, and enzymes), homeopathic medicine, exercise routines, and stress-reduction techniques.

All four Superwomen you read about suffered from chronic diseases caused by high stress, decreased immunity, and poor dietary choices, coupled with feelings of isolation, depression, anxiety, and unworthiness. In the next chapter, we'll tackle stress and how to mitigate its effects.

Before you turn the page, affirm for yourself:

I AM LOVED. I AM WELL. I AM GOD'S CHILD.

CHAPTER 4

The Stress of Racism and Food for All of Us

Why do we always try to please other people, take care of everything else, and let people walk over us?
It is time to stand up.

—Diane

Racism Is Alive and Well

STRESS is an underlying cause for many of our diseases. Racism is a cause for psychological stress associated with heart disease, infectious diseases, and inflammatory processes such as asthma and autoimmune diseases. Because of stress, we are dying faster and younger, and we're suffering more. Understanding the impact of stress and how to mitigate its effects is essential for health, wellbeing, and longevity.

Allow me to share a story with you. One day I asked my receptionist to call the next new patient on my schedule as she had not yet arrived. Cheryl came into my office to tell me the new patient was on the phone and was confused, even though she had returned my receptionist's call the day before to confirm the appointment. After we exchanged introductions, the woman explained that she had made the appointment for her son. She told me she got confused when Cheryl called the day before because she thought it was for another doctor with the same last name. And even though she called us back she did not realize the difference in phone numbers or addresses at the time of confirmation. She said when she called the other doctor's office that day, the receptionist there said they did not have a scheduled appointment. She did not think to call my office.

Part of it had to do with me, of course, and part of it was in the way she was explaining herself, and I was simply confused by what she was telling me. When I asked her to repeat herself, she changed her story. She said the other doctor's name was not the same as mine and the appointment was for her. Even though we were 45 minutes into the appointment time, I offered to allow her to come in immediately to begin the interview process, but she refused. She wanted to make another appointment and did not want to pay another deposit fee. I told her that, given the circumstances, I would not be willing to change the policy for her.

This woman suddenly became hostile over the phone. She began yelling and saying, "Who do you think you are?" I told her I was sorry for the confusion but was not willing to talk to her anymore if she was going to be offensive.

Ten minutes later her husband called back. He began the conversation by asking bluntly, "What have you done to my wife? She said you were rude and unpleasant to her."

I told him what happened and that his wife was already upset when we called her. I assured him I was neither rude nor unpleasant. He threatened me by telling me he knew a lot of people in Washington and he would see to it they would never come to my office. He also threatened to write to the Better Business Bureau. I told him I was sorry for the confusion and that he was entitled to do whatever he thought he should do.

Then it happened.

He said, "You're Black, aren't you? You're a Black doctor?"

I asked him what difference it made whether I was White or Black. Without answering me, he asked again and then he said, "I know you people, you Black doctors. You come from *nothing,* and think you are something. But you are *nothing* and you come from *nothing.*" Then he began to curse at me. I calmly told him I was not willing to engage in any further conversation with him and that I was hanging up the phone. And that's what I did.

Though I do not suffer from hypertension, I know my blood pressure was elevated. I could feel my face flushing with blood, and my heart racing, as if I were about to explode. I realized I was also shaking. I felt assaulted by the hatred in his voice and frightened by the evil of racism. I calmed down eventually, by thinking of my ancestors, even the ones I never knew, and knowing I did come from something.

I believe that because the stress, both overt and covert, of being Black in America is so permanent and consistent, the susceptibility to hypertension, for example, is constantly magnified. Over time the ability to normalize the pressure is lost without intervention.

With some understanding of stress, immunity and dis-ease, from the information that follows, we can see how the prolonged stress of racism, and our SAD (Standard American Diet) creates our susceptibility to dis-ease. In *A Path to Healing*, I wrote that racism is the most destructive and violent source of sickness and stress in America. It is woven into the historical fabric of this country, it shapes our behaviors and responses to life, and it invites stress to wreak havoc in our lives. We have all suffered from the institution of slavery. As a people, one people, our morals or standards with respect to right and wrong behavior have been reduced to a goal. Our passions—emotions and sexual desire/lust—dominate our reason and ethical principles. Just as African slaves taught their offspring, so the Caucasian masters taught theirs.

Slavery was the most demeaning act of humankind. In America, slavery was a well-designed, orchestrated system that resulted in the dehumanization and destruction of an entire ethnic group of people—in character, mind, body and spirit. Slavery created constant, obvious, immediate, and certain stress. These Africans, whose psyches were crippled, were responsible through the generations for our self-identity and socialization, our integrity, and self-esteem. Many people of color are still shackled by the chains of the past, the products of racism and discrimination.

Poverty is stressful. Lack of education is stressful. Job discrimination is stressful. Violence is stressful. Fear, depression, distrust, and isolation only encourage poor health habits. The daily burdens of living, for many African Americans, are stressful. As Opal Palmer Adisa writes in *Body and Soul: The Black Women's Guide to Physical Health and Emotional Well-Being* (1994), "Did you ever wonder why sisters look so angry? Why we walk like we've got bricks in our bags and will slash and curse you at the drop of a hat? It's because stress is hemmed into our dresses, pressed into our hair, mixed in our perfume, and painted on our fingers. Stress from the deferred dreams, the dreams not voiced; stress from always being at the bottom, from never being thought of as beautiful; stress from being a Black woman in America...." (p.369) (Villarosa L., 1994)[26]

Black women have been and still are the domestic support for the nation while we are routinely negated and neglected. Black women have had to care for children, grandchildren, parents, spouses, and in-laws. Several of my patients who have already transitioned (some in their 50s) spoke of raising children they didn't know their husbands had fathered during their marriage. And so, the stress continues.

The stress from racism and discrimination continues for many Caucasians, as well. All we need do is listen to the news for 15 minutes to hear about ethnic discrimination, murders of young Black men and women, White nationalism and supremacy groups on the rise, the attempts to take voting rights from African Americans, conspiracy theories about the politicians who seem to want a better America being pedophiles, the verbal and physical attacks on those politicians and their families, sexual harassment by White men, the denial of a legal election for President of the United States, and the subsequent violence at our Capitol, to understand the continuing effects of slavery—White supremacy and racism. And lest we forget the most recent assault upon and insult to all of us, when Ron DeSantis said that there was a benefit to slavery for African slaves, as they learned skills in how to be a blacksmith, for example.[27] Clearly his racism is being expressed in addition to his ignorance about history. The hatred is palpable and it is not new.

We are all affected by the dis-ease of racism. *The American Journal of Public Health* (May 2015), published a study conducted by The University of Pennsylvania. The conclusion was that all people regardless of ethnicity living in communities with high levels of racial prejudice were more likely to die younger than people living in more tolerant places. Yasmin Anwar reported research from UC Berkeley. "White Racism Linked to Fatal Heart Disease for Blacks and Whites" in *Berkeley News* 2016, has a similar conclusion, regarding Whites having racial bias and higher incidences of heart problems and circulatory disease.

In the wake of the murders of George Floyd, Breonna Taylor, Ahmaud Arbery, Michael Brown, Freddie Gray, and Sandra Bland (the list goes on and on), my patients ask, "What can we do?" For starters, begin using the word "ethnicity" and stop using the word "race." We are part of a global family; we are all children of God or whatever larger consciousness in which you believe. As I wrote in my first book, we are one race–HUMAN.

A Little History of "Race": It Is Not Real

"Race" is a man-made construct. It separates and divides us. The word didn't exist until 1580 and was then used only to denote certain groupings of people sharing physical characteristics and language. By the 18th century race was used for ranking the people of English colonies: Europeans, Amerindians, and Africans. The English had a long history of separating themselves from others and determining that those not from England were inferior. After failed attempts to conquer the Irish, the English turned to the Americas and its indigenous people. Subsequent wars, famine, and epidemics decreased the labor supply, creating a system of indentured servants, a system that was the precursor to North American slavery.

Some of the labor in the new world was initially performed by indentured servants. Some Africans were indentured, and they worked side-by-side with Whites. They worked together and rebelled together. The rebellions had to stop. It soon became obvious to the colonizers that European indentured servants were neither as strong nor as abundant as the African population.[28] They also knew that Africans cultivated crops and had skills necessary to build a new colony. The solution was to separate the Whites from the people of color.

And separate they did. The Virginia Slave Codes of 1705 were the culmination of laws passed from 1660 on and they cemented the fate of Africans in America. The code declared if a person was not Christian in their country of origin, they were a "slave." Africans, mulattos, and Indian slaves were considered property. The punishment for crimes, including leaving the plantation without written permission or associating with Whites, ranged from 60 lashes to having one's ears cut off to death. The law also stipulated that if an enslaver killed the person he'd enslaved while he was punishing him for a crime, the enslaver would not be criminally liable for murdering the enslaved person.

In justifying slavery, enslavers argued that Africans were inferior. It was at this time that "race" was used to sustain the inequality of Native Americans and Africans and continue to advance the idea of White supremacy. In 1830, a craniologist named Dr. Samuel Morton began measuring human skull sizes and determined that the skull size of White people meant they were the most intelligent race. East Asians ("Mongolians," as he called them), Southeast Asians, Native Americans, and finally Africans or "Ethiopians" followed. The slave masters quickly upheld this ideology. They received further support for their racist ideology in 1851 when an official from South

Carolina praised Morton for "giving to the Negro his true position as an inferior race." (Mitchell, 2018)[29]

These beliefs found their way into classrooms of universities. While studying for my PhD at the University of Pennsylvania in 1971, I had a professor of Criminology who made the statement to our class that the size of the Negro's brain was smaller than the brain of a White person and that is why Negroes are more prone to crime and violence. Dr. Morton, known as the father of scientific racism, made these claims before Charles Darwin's theory of evolution and before the discovery of DNA. Fortunately, a PhD student also at the University of Pennsylvania in 2018, Paul Wolff Mitchell, did his doctoral work on this subject noting that Dr. Morton did not consider body size. Brain and body size correlate and are adaptations to the climate in which people live. "From an evolutionary perspective there is no reason to suppose a link between cranial size and intelligence." He further says that the racial categories Dr. Morton suggests have no biological basis. (Mitchell, 2018)[30]

This sentiment was expressed in 2000 after genetic scientists gathered samples from people who self-identified as members of different races in order to create the first complete human genome. A pioneer of DNA sequencing, Craig Venter said at a White House ceremony that "the concept of race has no genetic or scientific basis." In 2019, the American Association of Physical Anthropologists Statement on Race and Racism was "the belief in 'races' as natural aspects of human biology and the structure of inequality (racism) that emerged from those beliefs are among the most damaging elements in the human experience, both today and in the past." (The Race Issue, 2018)[31] In America especially, because of slavery and miscegenation we are one race—HUMAN.

Over the last few decades genetic research has revealed that all humans are closely related, we all have the same collection of genes, and except for identical twins, we all have slightly different versions of them. All people alive today are Africans since we all evolved from

Homo sapiens in Africa. As we migrated, mutations and adaptations occurred that created changes in hair, skin color, lung capacity, blood type, etc.

So, I will say again, race is a man-made construct. It separates and divides us. We are one race, one people. Division by "race" is man's will, not God's will. It was and is still used to justify and explain the need for slavery. Racism is used for justifying and allowing the continuation of a system of inequality, injustice, and the accompanying self-degradation and demoralization of African Americans.

What Is the Effect of Stress on Our Bodies?

When we are stressed (emotionally), the sympathetic nervous system goes into the "fight or flight" response. The hypothalamus of the brain activates this response and triggers the pituitary gland (connected to the hypothalamus) to release adrenocorticotropic hormone (ACTH), which then triggers your adrenals (a gland that sits on top of each kidney) to produce cortisol. Blood vessels dilate and heart rates increase. When we cannot handle stress appropriately, our bodies continue to produce stress-inducing hormones. This leads to an increase in the production of adrenal hormones, like adrenaline, which affects blood pressure, and cortisol, which increases production of glucose (sugar). These reactions provide energy to large muscles, while reducing blood sugar utilization, and decreasing insulin sensitivity, all of which makes us more susceptible to hypertension and diabetes. Cortisol especially suppresses functions like your immune system response and digestion, and constrictsf the arteries, forcing the blood to pump harder.

Adrenaline (epinephrine) signals the body to increase heart rate and breathing and expands airways to push more oxygen into muscles. Blood vessels contract so that blood is sent to the heart and lungs, and non-essential functions (like digestion) are shut down. Chronic stress puts constant high levels of cortisol and adrenaline in your system, and chronic stress causes chronic inflammation. That is important because we now understand that inflammation is the basis of most dis-ease. Thus, stress is the basis of most dis-ease.

Many doctors use the term "immune system" as though most patients know exactly what it is and what it does. Allow me to explain and hopefully simplify. Your immune system is like a guard at the gate to keep danger away (e.g. bacteria, virus, or yeast). Actually, it is like many guards as there are many different types of cells that have this responsibility and are part of the immune system. The first line of defense and the first part of the immune system is the skin and mucous membranes. The skin (epithelial cells) has mucus cells that secrete a mucus-like substance that protects the body from assaults. Mucous membranes (also epithelial cells) line the inside of the body of the nasal passages, mouth, throat, lungs, down through the gastrointestinal/digestive system and the genitourinary system (the system that includes the kidneys, bladder, and all the organs involved with reproduction). Mucus is a sticky substance secreted by the cells of the mucous membrane that takes the bacteria, virus, or yeast into the digestive system where it is often destroyed.

If the bacteria, virus, or yeast continues to escape the first line of defense, continues to grow and multiply, the body secretes chemicals that alert the immune system that there is a problem. The body releases white blood cells, especially neutrophils, to attack the intruder. As the intruder is weakened and attacked, part of its body leaks out into the blood from the cell. These foreign parts are called antigens. The antigens come in contact with other white cells called lymphocytes and form antibodies to attack the intruders. All the while the invaders are also engulfed and digested by macrophages, another type of cell of the immune system, that manages to eliminate the foreign substance.

The immune system has many more parts and cells. What I have explained may assist you in understanding why it is so important to keep the system healthy and operating optimally. So, what is it that affects the immune system and depletes its ability to protect us?

Stress—in many forms, including mental, emotional, environmental, and dietary.

Stress inhibits the immune system's ability to destroy foreign microorganisms and hinders white blood cell function and production (white blood cells are necessary to fight infection). The parasympathetic nervous system, which is responsible for our bodily functions while we sleep, rest, and meditate, is also depressed during stress. It is responsible for stimulating digestion, and assisting with metabolism and relaxation. So with chronic stress, one can have exhaustion from trouble sleeping, headaches, dizziness, muscle tension, chest pain, stomach or digestive problems, diabetes, high blood pressure and heart problems, aches and pains, and depression and anxiety, all due to the depression of this system with the increased activity of the sympathetic system.

The level of stress we experience depends on how we respond to stimuli. Each of us develops different techniques to handle stress—exercise, meditation, sleep, vacations, yoga, etc. Also, individuals determine what is stressful or not. Stress can be caused by something minor for some, like speaking in public, an exam, sleep deprivation, or something profound, like the death of a loved one, divorce, or separating from a friend (romantic or platonic) or a family member.

In any instance, stress makes us more susceptible to spiritual, mental, emotional, and physical dis-ease as it suppresses our immune systems. One's susceptibility to disease changes as situations and circumstances change. Generally, the degree of immunosuppression is related to the level of stress. Through the relatively new discipline of psychoneuroimmunology (the study of how the mind and emotions affect the nervous and immune systems), mainstream medicine has finally acknowledged that there is a relationship between mind and body and that one may affect the other.

Emotional/mental stress can create habits that add more stress to the body, such as excess drinking, smoking, drug use (both prescribed and illegal) and poor food choices of increased sweets or salty foods. And there is other physical stress as well, when the body suffers a low blood sugar for example, that triggers an immune response and inflammation. And there is environmental stress from lack of healthy water choices, and airborne toxins. These circumstances come together to create all the diseases in chapter 1. In addition, poor maternal nutrition can lead to low-birth-weight babies, pregnancy-induced hypertension, and gestational diabetes, and subsequent chronic health problems. When life begins in this way it is difficult to create wellness. We must make different choices.

Stress and Inflammation

Chronic inflammation originates in the digestive system. What exactly is inflammation? To inflame is "to kindle or excite or arouse to a high degree of passion; to raise bodily tissue or blood to a feverish heat; to set aflame or afire," according to *Random House Webster's College Dictionary*. Inflammation is redness, swelling, and fever in the local area often with pain and disturbed function in reaction to an infection or physical or chemical injury. It is a normal response and evidence that the immune system is working effectively. The immune, hormonal, and circulatory systems are working to repair damaged tissue in the case of a scab forming after an injury, for example. The cells of the immune system are sent out to protect the body from a bacteria, virus, or fungus, as well as toxins or chemicals or any foreign particles.

Chronic inflammation produces free radicals which in turn produce more inflammation. Antioxidants are substances that protect your cells against free radicals. Free radicals are unstable atoms in the body that have one or more unpaired electrons in the form of oxygen, and they cause inflammation by damaging our cells. We get these unstable atoms in our bodies from the breakdown of certain foods.

Free radical damage is what occurs with every inhalation of a cigarette, by ingesting processed meats such as sausage, bacon, and salami that contain preservatives, refined carbohydrates and sugars, exposure to air pollutants, x-rays, industrial chemicals, mental/emotional stress, and cancer.

Much of our immune system cells are in the gastrointestinal tract (from our mouth to our anus). Many chronic metabolic conditions (increased blood pressure, high blood sugar, cholesterol, or triglycerides) are caused or influenced by chronic gut inflammation. When inflammation continues beyond its purpose of protection, and it is chronic from stress, the body has even higher levels of cortisol that will lead to more inflammation and a weakened immune system. Imagine your body being in a chronic state of inflammation- redness, and heat. Again, chronic stress creates chronic inflammation, causing flare ups of Rheumatoid Arthritis, Cardiovascular disease, depression and inflammatory bowel dis-ease.

Anti-inflammatory Supplements

In my practice I recommend several supplements to support the digestive system. I suggest that all patients take essential fatty acids and a probiotic daily. What is a probiotic? **Probiotics** are a group of good or friendly bacteria found in the gastrointestinal system (specifically esophagus, stomach, small and large intestine, colon) that aid in digestion. They are there as part of your normal bacteria and prevent the overgrowth of yeast and toxic bacteria, for example. There are trillions of them that work for our good. They also break down foods, manufacture some B vitamins, and help our immune system by accelerating the anti-inflammatory process. The two that are most beneficial are **Lactobacillus rhamnoses** and **Bifidobacterium lactis and longum**. (Be aware some yogurts do not include the Lactobacilli any longer and are full of sugar, as producers have found other bacteria to be better for mass production; read the labels).

Candida albicans, as it is called, is a common yeast in the intestine. However, it can overgrow in the GI tract if you take antibiotics too often and for a prolonged period or use oral birth control, or have too many sweets and white flour in your diet. Sugar inhibits the movement of macrophages/neutrophils, the cells that aid in the destruction of the bacteria/virus. You can get vaginal or oral yeast infections (thrush) if the yeast overgrows the normal/good bacteria of the GI tract. Supplementing daily with a probiotic replenishes the healthy, good bacteria for optimal gut health.

Reducing inflammation in the body is essential for good health. And there are supplements called essential fatty acids or **EFA's** such as omega 3 and omega 6 that have anti- inflammatory properties. They are essential for our health and yet we do not make them. Generally, EFA's make hormones that regulate the immune system and the central nervous system. Specifically, omega 6 oils contain GLA, or gamma-linolenic acid, which is converted to a hormone-like substance called prostaglandin. It is the varying types of prostaglandins that act as anti-inflammatory agents or pro-inflammatory agents.

DHA is the primary fatty acid in the brain and the retina of the eye. We get DHA before birth through the placenta and then through breast milk and, subsequently, diets of fish. You may have heard of fish oil, which also contains 2 types of omega 3 fatty acids, eicosatetraenoic acid (EPA) and docosahexaenoic acid (DHA). The omega 3 oils are quite beneficial for reducing inflammation in the gastrointestinal tract as well. They are found in salmon, sardines, herring, mackerel, cod (especially black cod), bluefish, lake trout, and tuna. Be mindful of tuna, however, as it tends to have higher levels of mercury than other fish, which can be toxic in excess.

Flaxseed also has alpha-linolenic acid (an omega 3 oil) that the body converts into **EPA** and **DHA**, the main fatty acids in fish oil. Also known as *Linum usitatissimum*, flax seed was likely first cultivated in Egypt. I ask my patients to use the omega 3 and 6 EFA, flaxseed, both ground (to put on top of oatmeal or pancakes for increased fiber) and whole (to be used in smoothies and blended with fruit). I suggest two to three teaspoons per day or, if it is oil, two capsules a day. They have been correlated with assisting with cardiovascular health, infant development, brain functioning, arthritis, hypertension, diabetes, and neurological support. Acting as a natural laxative, because it is so high in fiber, it's very beneficial for weight loss. Very often weight is waste. Flax seed actually contains two types of fiber, soluble and insoluble. Soluble fiber absorbs water in the intestine and slows down digestion, which may regulate blood sugar levels and lower cholesterol. The slower digestion also increases feelings of fullness and thus is important in weight loss. Insoluble fiber adds bulk to the stool and promotes bowel movements.

Flax seeds contain nutrients such as B vitamins and magnesium, and assist in lowering blood pressure. They are essential for anti-inflammation. I also suggest these supplements because of our SAD (standard American diet) which creates inflammation from free radical damage due to the chemicals, sugar, meats/animal fats, margarine, partially-hydrogenated vegetable oils, and processed foods in the American diet.

Borage oil is another type of omega 6 EFA that I ask my patients to use regularly as well, especially during the detox, as it has the benefit of reducing fat cravings and overeating. As an anti-inflammatory agent, I also use it for joint pain and eczema (topically and internally). It has one of the highest amounts of GLA of all the seed oils. It aids in controlling the release of molecules that are responsible for the body's inflammatory response. It is often used with Evening Primrose oil or fish oil for pain. It is also an antioxidant and lowers the oxidative damage that contributes to creating dis-ease. The plant, *Borago offficinalis,* is indigenous to North Africa and Europe.

Vitamin D3 is another nutrient that I suggest regularly because of its invaluable benefits to our bodies. It's actually not a true vitamin, but rather a hormone, because it can be made within our bodies by the skin's exposure to the sun. It is critical for building bones as it helps the body absorb and retain calcium. Equally as important it may prevent certain cancers like lung, colon, and prostate. Most people are deficient in vitamin D and our multivitamins are typically also deficient in the amounts provided. During the pandemic and beyond I recommend 2,000 IU of D3 a day. It has anti-inflammatory properties and it increases the function of immune cells, especially macrophages that protect against bacteria and viruses. Low levels are associated with a higher susceptibility to infection. In the gastrointestinal system, vitamin D3 assists in regulating inflammation and supporting the good bacteria.

Please do not think that taking the latest supplements while continuing a poor diet, having little sleep and exercise, and too much alcohol on the weekends to combat your stressful life will support your immune system. Supporting your system takes more effort than just taking supplements. They are called "supplements," not "food."

However, there are other supplements that would be helpful to combat the negative effects of stress and the damage created by free radicals. This free radical damage is a cause of inflammation and can be balanced by antioxidants (a substance that protects cells from the damage caused by free radicals) such as vitamin C and vitamin E. Other important substances which are not vitamins are carotenoids and flavonoid such as beta carotene and Quercetin, respectively.

Technically, all vitamins are manmade. They are not "natural." However, we need them. Let's begin with **vitamin C**. Without vitamin C for a period of three months, you may be prone to easy bruising, bleeding gums, weakness, fatigue, and an inability to heal wounds. This is a condition known as scurvy. The creation of scar tissue depends on collagen creation and the production of collagen depends on vitamin C. The strength of blood vessels, cartilage, and muscles also depends on vitamin C. Vitamin C is an important antioxidant as part of a basic regimen to prevent strokes, decrease inflammation, assist in cancer survival, and protect against bacterial and viral infections. It protects proteins in our body from free radical damage associated with infection. Vitamin C increases the lifespan of immune cells. Do not use chewable C, as it generally has too much sugar. and the time-release is unnecessary. The tablet of vitamin C may not dissolve, so use a capsule. I suggest 1,000 to 2,000 mg a day of buffered C for my patients.

Vitamin E neutralizes and scavenges the free radicals that damage our cells and protects the skin, especially from inflammation. It works best in conjunction with other anti-inflammatory nutrients, and helps to reduce heart disease by reducing blood fat levels and assists with menstrual cramps. It is also used topically for burns and scars from wounds. Excess vitamin E may increase blood pressure, however, so I never recommend more than 400 IUs daily.

Beta carotene is a carotenoid making carrots, cantaloupe, and sweet potatoes orange, peppers red, orange, and yellow, and collard greens, spinach, and kale green. Carotenoids are anti-oxidants and free radical scavengers. Beta carotene is a preformed vitamin A so one can take more of it than the vitamin itself, as vitamin A is toxic in high doses. Vitamin A is important for cell growth and maintaining healthy organs like the heart, kidneys, and lungs. It is also helpful for the skin and eyes. Beta carotene may reduce the risk of certain cancers such as lung (unless you are a smoker), breast and pancreatic.[32]

Quercetin, a flavanol and antioxidant found in plants and fruits, inhibits many steps in the proinflammatory cycle. It stabilizes cells and neutralizes inflammatory chemicals. Most importantly, it inhibits the release of histamine—a compound released by (mast) cells in response to injury and in allergic and inflammatory reactions. Histamine causes a runny nose or sneezing in response to an allergen. Flavonoids also protect collagen in the body. Collagen is necessary for the integrity of tendons and ligaments, and cartilage. Quercetin is most common in apples, onions, berries, cherries, and grapes.

While there are several minerals that are important for the body, I want to mention **zinc**, especially as we are continuing to be concerned about Covid-19. Zinc may lessen the potentially deadly symptoms of SARS-CoV-2 infection. Like the EFAs, it is essential, so although our bodies do not produce it naturally we must attain it through food or supplements. It is present in every cell and is a very abundant trace mineral. It supports the growth and normal functioning of immune cells, and is needed for the enzyme that makes our sense of taste and smell apparent. It also has a role in forming healthy skin, as it is needed for the formation of collagen in the skin. Zinc is important for reproductive (both male and female), digestive, eye, brain, and endocrine (e.g the thyroid) health. I recommend 25 mg daily. Zinc protects against free radical damage and acts synergistically with vitamin A in the transformation of lymphocytes into T cells that participate in the immune response by focusing on specific foreign particles. Zinc is also necessary for the production of digestive enzymes, especially for protein, called protease.

Please do not think you have to take all these supplements. They are, however, important for basic bodily function, even if you do not have any dis-ease. Based on your economic situation you will need to decide what to take. I do highly recommend C and D3 at minimum and eating fruits and vegetables, preferably organic, that are colorful and have texture.

Anti- inflammatory Herbs

My favorite anti-inflammatory herbs are *Boswellia scrrata* (Boswellia or Indian Frankincense), *Zingiber officinale* (Ginger), *Curcuma longa* (Curcumin), *Turmeric* which contains curcuminoids, the most effective of which is curcumin, and *Withania somnifera* (Ashwagandha).

Boswellia is native to Africa and India. It supports healthy inflammatory responses and blood circulation. The resin from the Boswellia tree has been used for centuries to treat chronic inflammatory conditions. I have used Boswellia effectively for both osteo and rheumatoid arthritis. Boswellic acid has been shown to suppress inflammation in the airways and inhibit secretions of certain substances that lead to inflammation, making it potentially useful for the treatment of asthma.

Ginger is used as a seasoning, and also for the treatment of nausea, vomiting,[33] and mild food poisoning. I suggest that patients grate ½ teaspoon of fresh ginger and steep it in a cup of hot water like a tea to relieve those symptoms. It is a natural anti-inflammatory agent, as it inhibits the inflammatory prostaglandins and other cells that create inflammation. It also has antioxidant properties. It is useful in the treatment of arthritis for pain relief, increased joint mobility, decreased swelling, and stiffness.

Curcuma longa (**curcumin**) is an antioxidant that neutralizes free radicals and stimulates other antioxidants. This herb inhibits the formation of cells, cytokines, that create inflammation. It is actually part of the ginger family. It may lower the risk of heart disease and play a role in fighting cancer cells.[34] Curcumin is useful as an anti-inflammatory nutrient in the treatment of arthritis, both osteo and rheumatoid.[35] It has antimicrobial (bacterial) and anti-cancer properties.

Withania somnifera, **Ashwagandha** or winter cherry, has been used for centuries in Ayurvedic medicine of India. It is also native to Africa and the Middle East. It has anti-inflammatory, anti-stress/anxiety, and sleep enhancing properties. The phytochemicals in Ashwagandha act as precursors to the hormones that regulate the stress response in the body. It has been shown to reduce cortisol, the stress hormone,[36] and therefore increase immune function. It reduces the activity of the hypothalamic-pituitary-adrenal (HPA) axis that regulates the stress response. It increases the activity of the killer cells that fight viruses. It is also useful for pain relief and decreasing the joint and muscle stiffness of osteoarthritis.[37] Taken along with resistance training, muscle strength and growth can increase.[38]

Allium sativa (**garlic**) is a great natural antibiotic, antiviral, and antifungal herb. It is used regularly to lower blood pressure and cholesterol, especially the bad cholesterol LDL, to prevent cardiovascular disease.[39] Garlic has antioxidant properties that guard against oxidative damage (free radicals) of cells. The sulfur compounds in garlic have detoxifying qualities for heavy metals like lead.[40] Be mindful it can thin the blood, so talk to your naturopathic physician if you are on blood thinners before taking it in pill form.

However you can combine curcuma, ginger and garlic along with onions, in heated oil before stir-frying or sauteing vegetables for a boost in immunity and a tasty, healthy meal.

The Stress of Foods

Inflammation is also linked to the stress of food allergies from milk, specifically casein, and gluten in wheat. Oils found in fast foods are also problematic—sunflower, corn, soy, peanut, safflower, and corn oils can cause negative responses in the body. (Olive, avocado, and grapeseed are better choices).

While I will talk more about diet and inflammation in chapter 6, I want to share some patients' food diaries with you to give you an example of the stress of foods and how it causes inflammation. For breakfast, a patient had coffee, Cheez-It crackers, Coco Puffs and cow's milk or Cap'n Crunch and cow's milk. And still others may have pork bacon and eggs, with grits and hash browns. Lunch is Boston baked pork and beans and a salad with iceberg lettuce, and dinner may be a salad with avocado dressing and more Cheez-Its. And there are those who have no breakfast, just coffee, with spinach and cheese ravioli for lunch with Chips Ahoy cookies. Dinner is a Subway sandwich with cold cuts.

Let's look at what these patients are really eating. The ingredients in Cheez-Its include TBHQ, soy, soybean/palm or canola oil, and skim milk. TBQH is tertiary butylhydroquinone, a Thai food additive designed to preserve food and keep it from changing color, thereby increasing its shelf life. It's found in noodles, crackers, and other fast and frozen food products. It is also in paint, varnishes, and skin care products. I generally tell patients if you cannot pronounce it you should not be eating it, and it would be better if you ate the packaging, not the product. TBQH has been connected to liver enlargement[41] and neurotoxic (brain and nervous system) disorders. Preservatives are not recognized as food, because they are not food. Since the body cannot get nutrients out of them and does not know what to do with them, it turns them into fat. Additives can increase hormones that are associated with an increased risk of obesity and diabetes.

What about Chips Ahoy cookies? Those ingredients listed are wheat, sugar, dextrose (which is another name for sugar), milk, sugar again, canola oil, palm oil, sugar again, high fructose corn syrup (which is another name for sugar), molasses (sugar), caramel (sugar), color, and artificial flavor. The chapter on nutrition will speak to the ills about cow's milk and sugar. Suffice it to say the other ingredients such as palm oil (which is high in saturated fat and clogs arteries), high fructose corn syrup (the number one causative factor for diabetes), and artificial flavors (causative factors for allergic reactions, food sensitivity, and digestive issues) are not particularly nutritious either. These are not "foods" as described in chapter 2 that promote growth and maintain life. They are foods that stress the body and further turn us to sand.

It's more than enough! Do not allow food to create even more damage.

We have been victimized sufficiently by the system, our families and ourselves. We have been marginalized, discounted and reduced, as was intended by the three-fifths clause in the Constitution that labeled enslaved African people only three-fifths of a person.

So, declare boldly:

I AM LOVED. I AM WELL. I AM GOD'S CHILD.

MORE

A greater or additional amount of something; in greater quantity, amount, increase, degree or measure.

ENOUGH!

Adequate for the want or need; sufficient for the purpose or to satisfy desire; to express impatience or exasperation.
    Synonyms—plenty

CHAPTER 5

Do Something Different / Take Control

Oh, de people never didn't' put much faith to de doctors in dem days, mostly, dey would use de herbs in de fields for dey medicine.

—Josephine Bacchus, 81-year-old ex-slave from Marion, South Carolina

Colored folks were brought up on these old home remedies. Like I tell you 'bout this fever grass hump. You know when folks in the community—lots of 'em would make that fever grass the same day or night and give it to 'em. You know we stayed up too, with the chillun; didn't have no doctors. These old home remedies; that's all I ever took. Right now, you know, I ain't never been to a doctor.

—Mildred Graves, 84, Macon County, Alabama

Naturopathic Medicine

It happens all the time in my practice: African American patients, when pondering my prescription for herbs, recount how a grandmother or aunt or great uncle used herbal remedies. For precisely what condition of the body or spirit, or what herbs exactly, patients usually don't know or can't remember. But they remember relatives taking these natural remedies as their primary form of medicine.

This doesn't surprise me. For years I was vaguely aware of a certain "yellow bush" my grandmother told me her mother boiled and dispensed to her children for colds and influenza. But I never knew the name of this magical shrub. Was it chamomile, a medicinal herb used by ancient Egyptians and Greeks? (It is recorded that Hippocrates is the Father of Modern Medicine. However, like so much of history, the accomplishments of people of color are not included. Imhotep, a Black Egyptian, was practicing and writing about medicine 2,200 years before Hippocrates). Or perhaps it was *Hydrastis*, commonly known as golden seal, which is widely recognized today as one of the most popular and effective antibacterial herbs?

Our knowledge of herbal medicine in this country is a direct, wondrous gift from African slaves and early American Indians (Lumbee and Cherokee tribes, in particular). Yet millions of Americans today remain profoundly estranged from it.

Call it folk medicine. Call them home remedies. Now, however, through more research and colleges and universities offering degrees in naturopathic medicine, it's not simply folk medicine or home remedies. We know of it only through oral histories preserved through the ages. This is particularly true of elderly Blacks living in the South. Many of them still use herbal medicine as their main source of care or as a supporting treatment. In a conversation that I had with my sociology professor, Dr. Wilbur Watson, while in undergraduate school, he said the Black elderly are put off by the impersonal treatment of the current medical system, with its endless lists of doctor referrals and specialists for virtually every organ. In my current practice I find that not much has changed.

But the use of herbal medicine in American history is still, by and large, ignored by the medical establishment. Older African Americans in the South, as well as those who have lived for decades in racially segregated neighborhoods, depend more on traditions and the wisdom of their elders than on conventional medicine. There is a belief that in rural communities, traditional medical practices should not be violated. And there are limits on how much technology will be accepted. Advancements in medical tools and techniques may complement the existing traditional system, but not replace it.

The Black elderly have purposely shrouded their customs in secrecy for fear of being ridiculed or misunderstood. Similarly, when many of my patients tell other doctors they are seeing a naturopathic physician, they usually receive a snicker, dismissive gesture, or a negative comment.

For a complete discussion of the beginnings of naturopathic medicine in the US during slavery, see chapter 2, "Naturopathy: The Roots" in my first book, *A Path to Healing: A Guide to Wellness for Body, Mind, and Soul*. (Sullivan, 1999)[42]

Some of what you are about to read is found in my first book, referenced above. I have come to understand, over the years, that learning requires repetition. Some of us need to have this information repeated again and again. We learn when we are ready to learn. Not before.

So, what is naturopathic medicine? How does it work? What can it do for you? How does it differ from conventional, or allopathic, medicine? Why does it play such a crucial role in the wellbeing of black women?

Health is freedom from spiritual, mental, emotional, and physical limitations. Spiritual and mental freedom is the ability to express oneself creatively without egocentrism and to think clearly with compassion and will. Emotionally healthy people are free to experience a wide range of feelings: grief, anger, anxiety. They are able to feel these emotions and yet detach from them, maintaining an underlying sense of inner peace and balance. Not dwelling on any one emotion, they leave themselves open to the next moment and they experience the fullness of life.

Creating good health is not the responsibility of the doctor or pharmaceutical companies as conventional medicine has led us to believe. Good health is our individual responsibility. Because of the stress of certain lifestyles, unhealthy foods, and negative thought patterns, most of us are functioning below zero on a health scale of one to ten. My job is to assist people in getting back up to one using homeopathy, nutrition and herbs so they can support themselves through the rest of their healing process. The patient and I are in a partnership that involves changing his/her lifestyle. The patient does the work as well as the healing. I am simply the facilitator who believes in the body's ability to be well given the proper support. I tell my patients they cannot drop their body off and pick it up at five o'clock like a car. They must get involved with their healing.

While my medical training in the basic sciences as a naturopathic student was the same as that of someone in allopathic medical school, my philosophy about health was and is still very different. My philosophy about health is based on principles of vitalism.

Allopathic vs. Naturopathic Philosophy

Naturopathic medicine (which is complementary medicine, not alternative) is based on the philosophy of vitalism. Vitalism maintains that life is more than a complex series of chemical and physical reactions. It relies on a belief that there is a soul, that which makes us breathe, that coordinates and organizes these chemical reactions. This force allows an organism to develop, reproduce, and repair itself.

In allopathic medicine, symptoms of disease are thought to be a result of a physiological reaction to bacteria or virus and symptoms are considered destructive and must be controlled or eliminated so that order can be restored. When the symptoms disappear, it is assumed that the disease has been eradicated or at least controlled.

Naturopaths believe that the symptoms of a disease are not solely the result of a bacteria or virus, but that they are the body's intelligent response to a causative agent, stress, bacteria, or virus. Symptoms are indicators of the body's attempt to eradicate a harmful agent, bacteria, or virus. Symptoms reflect the innate intelligence of an organism to maintain wellness.

When drugs are given, they work against the body's attempt to heal itself. There certainly are times when bacteria must be destroyed rapidly and mechanical intervention, or surgery, is necessary. However, the body needs to be supported in its effort to increase resistance and decrease susceptibility. Drugs relieve symptoms, but they don't stimulate our body's natural ability to heal. And they can produce undesirable effects. One example is the rampant use of prophylactic antibiotics for children with ear infections. Antibiotics eliminate lactobacillus acidophilus, the body's normal bacterial flora. Once eliminated, yeast is allowed to flourish in the intestines, and this causes diarrhea and nausea. Without proper support for the body, the earaches reoccur and so do the antibiotic prescriptions. This, of course, leads to an ongoing cycle.

This is not to say that naturopathy does not at times support the use of drugs in some situations. But the use of natural therapies means there is little suppression of the immune system and therefore few unintended effects. Naturopathic remedies work to strengthen and support the body's innate healing power.

The first tenant of the naturopathic physician's oath is "to do no harm." The oath continues with the following: to act in cooperation with the healing power of nature, to address the fundamental cause of disease, to heal the whole person through individualized treatment, to teach the principles of healthy living and preventive medicine, and to practice prevention with patients and the public.

Differing Perspectives of Health

Because of underlying differences in their philosophies, allopaths and naturopaths (including homeopaths), view health from different perspectives. Allopaths have a philosophy of illness. Some have changed their views and their practices. Most base their understanding of sickness on the germ theory. They believe bacteria or viruses cause disease and that symptoms are the disease itself. It is not until the symptoms localize to a specific organ that allopaths classify and diagnose the disease. They usually treat the disease with drugs or surgery and measure the success of the treatment when the symptoms go away. Oftentimes, success is achieved by any means necessary, no matter how dangerous the drug.

Naturopathic medicine focuses on health and wellness. Naturopaths are concerned about the health of your body and what defenses your body is using to create wellness. We are concerned about maintaining wellness, not just fighting illness. We determine your wellness through conversation, by noting your emotional, spiritual, and physical well-being, and by assessing risk factors such as social and emotional stress and nutritional deficiencies. As a classical homeopathic physician, I want to know the stresses in your life, issues, and challenges you have had to overcome and what effect you believe those challenges had on your body, mind, and emotions. I want to know your fears, sleep patterns, and food cravings as well. For example, I may ask you why you believe you have this condition? What was occurring in your life at the time of or five years before the onset of the disease? What makes you angry or sad and what is your behavior when you are angry or sad? What is your experience of anger? Or are you impatient or irritable? Because we know that a change in one part of the body creates change in another, we must study the whole organism.

Our bodies strive to maintain homeostasis. Homeostasis is defined as the maintenance of stability and constancy while adapting to changes. Symptoms signal a disturbance, instability or an undesired change in the body. Complementary medicine practitioners appreciate symptoms because they are signs the body is creating resistance to a stressor like, for example, bacteria. A symptom is not a disease or the cause of a disease, but rather the body's way to defend itself and keep itself well. A symptom is the best reaction your body can make when it encounters bacterial, viral, or psychological stressors. The body's only job is to keep itself well. When treating a sick patient, naturopaths attempt to stimulate the body's ability to respond to the offending agent and repair itself. Fever, for example, is a symptom all of us are familiar with. A fever is an important defense mechanism which stimulates the body's white blood cells and interferon secretions, both of which help fight infections. Eliminating the fever with a drug suppresses the body's natural defenses and prevents it from fighting off the underlying cause of the fever.

Let me offer some food for thought: have you ever gotten a headache from a lack of aspirin in your body? No. Headaches can result from a lack of sleep, constipation, dehydration, a food allergy or too much computer screen time, but never from a lack of aspirin. Similarly, do you get GERD from a lack of Zantac? Does high cholesterol occur because you haven't had enough Lipitor? In both cases, no. These conditions result from our lifestyle choices. The conventional medical establishment supports the devaluation of health and wellness via their diagnoses, caused by poor habits, stresses, and lifestyle and prescribes medication to treat the problem.

Rather than attempting to control the disease or wiping out the symptom, naturopaths work to support and strengthen the body's natural healing ability and decrease susceptibility. Naturopaths refer to susceptibility as the organism's degree of strength against offending agents. Susceptibility is determined by levels of mental, emotional, and physical stress.

The most recent Coronavirus pandemic more severely impacted those whose immune systems were weakened by other dis-eases like diabetes, hypertension, and heart disease and therefore, unable to respond effectively to the virus.

Lifestyle Changes

Naturopathic medicine seeks to normalize bodily functions, restore a state of wellness, and prevent disease. The philosophy of *vis medicatrix naturae,* the healing power of nature, is fundamental to naturopathic medicine. Using everything nature provides, I cooperate and support the body's innate ability to heal itself. As a naturopath, I avoid the use of drugs and procedures that interrupt normal functioning and have unintended negative side effects. I use nontoxic therapies based on physiologic principles to treat the whole individual, not just the disease or condition, because the whole person is involved in the healing process. My concern is with the cause, treatment, and prevention of disease.

One of the most important, if not the most important aspect of my work is listening to the patient. Patients are not just heart disease, diabetes, hypertension, lupus, or cancer. They have stories, too often stories of abuse—sexual, physical, mental, and/or emotional from the alcoholic father/mother or the absent, distant, or fearful father/mother—and this cycle of abuse continues into adulthood and marriage. They speak of self-deprecating behaviors and just never being good enough. They tell me of their anxiety from an early age when their parents fought or their siblings committed suicide. I listen with compassion, humility, and caring as I allow this human to tell their story and feel honored that they have chosen me. The value of listening is not only to begin to understand the patient. It is also to allow the patient to hear themselves and learn what may have triggered their body to respond with dis-ease, thus providing awareness that can be used for healing. Listening of course also fosters trust and feelings of being heard and cared about.

Naturopathic doctors teach patients to make lifestyle changes that focus on proper nutrition, elimination, or reduced use of drugs and alcohol, stress reduction, exercise, rest, meditation, yoga, and recreation. As you will read in subsequent chapters, in addition to a homeopathic remedy, my patients are given strategies for being responsible for their health, such as dietary recommendations, stress reduction techniques, and botanical (herbal) and vitamin prescriptions for their wellness. I am a primary care physician working in concert with patients to establish good health habits.

Naturopathic philosophy believes that whatever is going on inside and outside your body can minimize or maximize health. Most dis-ease begins because of a violation of healthy living. Healthy living includes eating natural unprocessed foods, getting adequate rest and exercise, having a positive attitude, staying hydrated, living a moderately-paced lifestyle, and avoiding excess alcohol, drugs, and polluted environments. Unfortunately, for many African Americans, especially women, life precludes healthy living, giving way to unhealthy lifestyles and habits. Benedict Lust, who brought naturopathy to the United States in 1902, wrote the following in his first editorial in the *Naturopathic and Herald of Health* (1902): "We plead for the renunciation of poisons from the coffee, white flour, glucose (sugar), lard (pork fat) and like venom of the American table to patent medicines, tobacco, liquor, and other inevitable recourse of perverted appetite. We long for a time when an eight-hour day may enable every worker to stop existing long enough to live; when the spirit of universal brotherhood shall animate business and society and the church...when people may stop doing and thinking and being for others and be for themselves...." In other words, take care of yourself so that you can take care of others.

The scope of naturopathy is broad because we treat people, not diseases or organ systems. Every phase of life is important to the naturopath. We treat everyone from the infant to the elderly using therapies such as homeopathy, nutrition, botanicals (herbs), acupuncture, hydrotherapy, exercise, manipulation, and massage. Our specialties then are in the treatments we use and not necessarily in organ systems such as the heart, cardiology, joints, or rheumatology as in conventional medicine since the organs are not separate from the soul. Most recently, however, there are naturopaths who specialize in pediatrics, oncology, endocrinology, and gastroenterology.

As Lust said in 1902: "In a word, naturopathy stands for the reconciling, harmonizing, and unifying of nature, humanity and

God. Fundamentally therapeutic because men need healing; elementally educational because men need teaching; ultimately inspirational because men need empowerment; it encompasses the realm of human progress and destiny." (Lust, 1937)[43.]

Dr Lust was constantly fighting to advance naturopathy, the term he used to describe the integration of botanical (herbal) medicine, homeopathic medicine, nutritional and lifestyle guidance, as well as acupuncture and chiropractic medicine. The conventional medical establishment continually attempted to shut down the schools that taught and offices of those practicing our science and art. Discriminated against at every turn, he was arrested nearly 20 times over his career, as he fought for a marginalized profession.

The American Medical Association (the organization for the allopathic or conventional doctors) spearheaded additional discrimination against African American doctors and women by not allowing them to be a member of the organization for 100 years. Ultimately the conventional medical establishment, through the Flexner Report (1910), was successful in closing five African American medical schools[44] as well as schools for naturopathy. The only African American schools that remained open were Howard University College of Medicine and Meharry Medical College. African Americans, especially in the South continued their involvement in herbal medicine, a forerunner of naturopathy.

Botanical (Herbal) Medicine

During the past several decades we have seen a resurgence of naturopathic medicine. I say resurgence because naturopathy is not new. Though naturopathic medicine has been around for centuries, many people, especially African Americans, have not taken full advantage of this heritage. If you haven't, it may be time to start.

Naturopathy is the medicine of the past, and part of our heritage that we share with the indigenous people of this country, as some herbs used today were the same herbs brought to the Caribbean and the South during the slave trade and used by African slaves. It was not until 12 years after my graduation from Bastyr University that I learned about the role and contributions of African slaves in the development of naturopathy. Like much of our history, this too was not a part of our learning. Specifically, some of the families of plants that slaves used and we use today are from West Africa, Mauratania, a country bordered by Senegal, Morocco, Algeria, and Mali.

Though the families of plants were very similar, enslaved Africans had to familiarize themselves with the geography, topography, and species of plants of the West Indies for survival. And they did just that.

Unfortunately. the process of recognizing and replacing the herbs in formulas or as a single herb for curative purposes was mostly verbal and passed on from generation to generation by the same method, as slaves were forbidden to read and write. Naturopaths are the beneficiaries of herbal medicine. For example, *Strychnos Nux vomica* was used as a poison and is now used homeopathically for alcohol poisoning or a hangover from drinking too much alcohol. *Rauwolfia seroentina* was used as a tranquilizer and for hypertension. *Euphorbia* is, homeopathically and as an herbal preparation, used for relief of colds and breathing disorders like asthma and bronchitis. *Marrubium vulgare* or Horehound was also a favorite for bronchitis and is still very useful. I use all these plants today in my practice.

The *Asteraceae* family of plants is also full of herbs that we use today: arnica, a wonderful homeopathic remedy for bruising, falls, and any injury; *Matricaria chamomilla* which you may have used as a tea for a restful sleep; *Arctium lappa* or Burdock, which can be eaten or consumed as a tea as well and is used for detoxification, especially for the liver; *Taraxacum officinale* or dandelion is often put in salads or prepared as a tea for liver and anti-inflammatory support; and *Achillea millefolium* or yarrow, when mixed with *Euphrasia officinalis*, or eyebright, *Armoracia rustcana*, commonly known as horseradish, and *Mahonia aquifolium*, which is Oregon grape is a great combination to relieve symptoms from allergies. DO NOT TAKE THESE HERBS WITHOUT THE ADVICE OF A NATUROPATHIC PHYSICIAN OR AN HERBALIST. IF YOU DO TAKE THEM AND DO NOT RECEIVE THE INTENDED RESULT IN THREE MONTHS, PLEASE CONTACT A HEALTH PROFESSIONAL. DO NOT TAKE IF PREGNANT WITHOUT THE ADVICE OF A NATUROPATHIC PHYSICIAN.

The most common traditional medicine across the continent of Africa is herbal medicine. This is the case for many reasons—both historical and contemporary, given the inadequate or non-existent health care in the continent (similar also in areas of the United States).

The distrust of the European doctors and their aggressive treatments also led the slaves to prefer their traditional plant medicine rather than conventional medicine. Many slaves were "secret doctors," called such because they would be asked to treat another slave or the master's family with herbs. The master could not afford to lose a slave through the harsh treatments of conventional doctors such as leeching, bloodletting, or giving toxic doses of mercury and antimony.

In his book *Roll Jordan Roll* (1974), Eugene Genovese remarks how one planter, John Hamilton of Williamsport, Louisiana, wrote in a letter to his brother about his use of slaves for treatment. "I am sorry to learn that you have been unfortunate with the Negroes. Your doctors are rather a rough set—they give too much medicine. It's seldom that I call upon a physician. We doctor upon the slaves and have first rate luck."

Fanny Kemble, a slave owner's wife, is said to have written in her journal about one slave's gift of healing. "I was very sorry not to ascertain what leaves she had applied to her ear. These simple remedies, resorted to by savages, and people as ignorant are generally approved by experience, and condescendingly adopted by science."

The preference for medicinal plants was also because of familiarity, and because the healer offered counseling and looked at the whole person, not just the symptoms. Just as naturopaths and homeopaths investigate the cause of illness with the focus on a patient's lifestyle, habits, stress, and relationships, African healers considered the environment, family, and circumstances. They pursued the cause.

Now here in America, African Americans are often distrustful of conventional medicine and the endless list of drugs, specialists, and surgeries needed. Sometimes when I ask a patient why they have come to me, they will say, "they are trying to kill me with all these medicines, doc."

Diet was also important. In West Africa the diet was simple and nutritious: yams, okra, black eyed peas, grains, roots, vegetables, and fruits. Yams are high in beta carotene, an antioxidant that gives the yam its color. Antioxidants prevent something called free radical damage, which is damage to cells that cause inflammation, cardiovascular disease, and cancer, for example. As mentioned in the chapter on Stress, free radical damage is what occurs with every inhalation of a cigarette, exposure to air pollutants, x-rays, industrial chemicals, mental/emotional stress, and cancer.

Black eyed peas and other beans are high in fiber and other nutrients like copper, folate (folic acid needed for healthy red blood cells, pregnancies and fetal development), and iron needed for oxygen transport and DNA (the substance that carries out the instructions for your development, functioning and growth—our genes). Africans did not come here eating salt-laden fast foods, fatback, and pig's feet. Our ancestors' health habits and lifestyle were very different before coming to America. We must make different choices.

Naturopathy is stronger than ever at the moment, with five accredited universities in the US and two in Canada, because this medicine is the medicine of the future. Thomas Edison said in 1903, "The doctor of the future will give no medicine, but will interest his patient in the care of the human frame, in diet and in the cause and prevention of disease."

We need a true health care system, not a continuation of the sick care system. Linda Villarosa, in her book, *Under The Skin: The Hidden Toll of Racism on American Lives and On the Health of our Nation*, says: "Our nation, even with the most expensive health-care system and arguably the best medical technology in the world, cannot rely only on clinical and technical solutions to dig our way out of the nation's most vexing health issues, which include high rates and infant and maternal mortality and lowered life expectancy compared with other wealthy countries as well as persistent racial disparities in nearly every health outcome. Without a personal connection to offset the largely impersonal nature of the current medical system, spending more money on health care will never erase the problems dogging America or close the racial gap. Our country must instead combine the rigorous science and advanced technology we are known for with kindness, care, and support." (Villarosa L., 2022)[45]

Homeopathy Medicine

Whether an acute or chronic condition, homeopathy considers the whole person. It is not enough to ask a person about the specifics of a headache, but we also need to know the mood and temperament of the person, their sleep patterns, anxieties, and concerns (stresses) during and before the onset of an illness, food cravings, the state of their memory and concentration, and their fears, for example. I am treating a person who happens to have headaches, not the headache.

This treatment of the whole person was the result of human experimentation, which was essential for Dr. Hahnemann, the founder of homeopathy. In 1796, he was disillusioned by the practice of allopathic medicine and left his medical practice in order that he would "do no harm." At the time quinine, which is extracted from cinchona bark, was used to treat malaria. There was much discussion among his peers as to how quinine was working. He took cinchona bark repeatedly in toxic amounts and created the symptoms of malaria. He then, along with his colleagues, tested many different substances from nature by giving the substances in toxic amounts to healthy subjects, and recorded all the effects, physical, mental, and emotional. *These effects reflected the curative potential of the substance because the effects of the toxicity were the same as the expressions of the dis-ease they were trying to heal.* Healthy subjects were given a natural substance in high (toxic) enough concentration to disturb their well-being and stimulate their defense mechanism. The body's response (vital force/the energy of the immune system) to this foreign substance was the most intelligent response it could make at the moment, and that response was known as symptoms. The healing substance had to produce the same signs and symptoms, when given to a well person in a toxic amount. This systematic process of testing substances on healthy people is called "proving."

Dr. Hahnemann then created a Materia Medica with the information from the provings by cataloging and recording the therapeutic properties of every substance he and his colleagues tested. They recorded all the mental symptoms (mood, fears/phobias, delusions) and sleep patterns exhibited from being given the poisonous doses, as well as how every organ was affected by the plant, mineral, or animal substance. Food cravings and aversions, along with foods that disagreed with the person, were also recorded.

Being a physician and chemist, Dr. Hahnemann understood that, in order to affect the vital force (energy), a substance's energy must be compatible with that of the vital force. He knew he had to provide energy to the defense mechanism to help it maintain balance and wellness. Hahnemann used his provings to determine which substances would match the same signs and symptoms exhibited by the defense mechanism at the time of dis-ease. He had to find a way to make the concentration of the material substance non-toxic to avoid increasing the patient's illness. Finally, after much trial-and-error, Hahnemann discovered that by diluting and shaking the substance he could increase the material's intensity (energy) and make it available to the defense mechanism. A substance that was diluted and shaken had a greater therapeutic result and had virtually no toxic risk. Hence the name homeopathy – *homeo* means same, and *pathos* means suffering; so, it is to heal the suffering with something that is the same, also known as the "Law of Similar."

Thankfully, Dr. Hahnemann's work did not end with his death in 1843. Internationally, homeopathy is the second most used medical system according to the World Health Organization. I've been blessed to study with some of the best homeopaths in the world. More than 25 years ago I began studying with Indian homeopaths, specifically Rajan Sankaran in Mumbai, India. India's use of homeopathy dates to before 1881 when the first Homeopathic Medical College was founded in Calcutta. Now more than 100 million people use homeopathy exclusively and there are about 200,000 registered homeopaths in India.

I understood from past educational experiences and degrees that we respond to our individual perceptions of circumstances and not to the events themselves. These perceptions are what we call stress. And we respond to life based on these perceptions, also known as delusions in homeopathy. We form ideas and ideologies about life and view the world through those perceptions or experiences. It is our individuality.

The stress is an experience, however, not just cause and effect. From Dr. Sankaran I have learned that that experience produces a sensation that encompasses the whole person. It is not confined to the mind and body and therefore not specifically human. He writes in *The Other Song*, "It is an experience the human shares with animals, plants, and minerals and the things that make up this earth." (Thomson Press, India 2008, p.54) We each have a spirit in us as a result of some life stressors. When that spirit that we have borrowed from nature, for a survival mechanism, becomes more demanding and visible without a path for expression, it is suppressed and crystallizes as a physical, mental, and emotional pathology.

Dr. Sankaran states further, "... the non-human melody expressed in the human can best be heard through the language of disease. And the language of disease in a person can be heard in the way he voices his complaints, the exact sensation of his aches and pains or other complaints. It can also be seen in his perception of his situation, the words used to describe it, and the effect of the situation on him coupled with his reaction to that situation."

Though I cannot give all the information in the provings/Materia Medica for the remedies prescribed for Diane, Darlene, Mary, and Letitia, I can share some of the reasons they received a particular remedy. You read in the chapter on stress how we are affected by situations we perceive as stressful. When the stress hormones are released, those hormones affect our physical body and activate genes that create dis-ease.

Diane perceived and experienced her mother's displeasure of her such that she did not like her mother and was certain her mother did not like her, but rather tolerated her, especially after her father became ill. I gave her a mineral salt called *Natrum muriaticum.* She believed her experience of an early pregnancy and subsequent marriage upset her parents and turned them against her. The separation from her child's father and the heartbreak she felt cemented Diane's feelings that she had to be independent and could no longer trust. These experiences presented as suppression of grief, disappointment in love, heartbreak, and betrayal. She thought often of her past and would dwell on negative experiences. She had become a loner and cried alone at home fearing it would otherwise be seen as weakness. She didn't trust anyone enough to let them into her inner world. She had very few friends and no close friends. Her physical dis-ease was a result of her immune system responding to the stress of these experiences. Had I given the mineral salt to a well person in a toxic amount, I could create these feelings and sensations.

Remember Darlene? The remedy I prescribed for her is called *Ignatia amara. Ignatia amara* is a plant, because she had the experience of all the responses of the vital force that I know from the provings. Specifically, the irritability, impatience, sighing, wanting to be alone, having the sensation of a "hole" (void) in her heart, and the sensation the heart is torn or was ripped out after experiencing all of the deaths in her family. She also expressed guilt and was weeping during our session even though the deaths had happened more than a year ago—some more than five years ago. This was her experience of grief. You cannot touch grief, guilt, a void, or a torn heart. These sensations are all energy. These symptoms are not palpable.

If I were to give a toxic, poisonous amount of the plant ignatia to a well person, I could create these symptoms, sensations, and feelings even though the person had not experienced death of a loved one, shock, or a bad break up. The toxicity could create a nervous, sensitive, moody, melancholic temperament. The remedy is not the actual toxic substance, but rather a diluted substance or the energy of the plant *Ignatia amara*. The energy of the remedy is stronger than the energy Darlene's defense mechanism created in response to the experience of grief and was able to remove the energy of the defense mechanism. Hence, "Like cures like." As I mentioned previously, *homeo* means the same and *pathos* means suffering. We are healing the suffering with something that is similar or the same.

Mary was given the mineral remedy *Argentum nitircum* for the sensation that things were out of control. Like so many women of color, Mary grew up with an alcoholic father who abused her mother. There was constant chaos and craziness in the house. She felt trapped and helpless. Mary's reaction of panic attacks, feelings of overwhelm, uncertainty, and anxiety, as well as her physical symptoms, were a direct result of her reactions to these events. She had fears of heights and was claustrophobic, because she was fearful of anything that made her feel out of control of her environment. She told me that she remembers attending a school for "Colored Students" and seeing the signs pointed toward the school for "Whites Only." She said, "When we went into town we could buy from the establishment, but [we] had to go in the back door. When we went to the doctor, we had to go in the back door. It was how we grew up. I felt we didn't matter.

We were the underdog. I felt worthless [and] less than...."

Argentum nitricum is silver nitrate and is considered a poison when ingested. It is corrosive and can cause potentially fatal gastroenteritis and gastrointestinal bleeding. As a homeopathic remedy I have given it many times to people who have acid reflux along with the other sensations of being out of control and associated fears/phobias. (Interestingly, silver nitrate used to be used in the eyes of newborns in the early 1900s to prevent any neonatal eye infections and blindness from Neisseria gonorrhoeae.)

If I were to give a toxic amount of the mineral *Argentum nitricum* to a well person, the toxicity would bring about the sensations of panic, overwhelm, anxiety, helplessness, life being out of control, with not enough time to accomplish tasks, and resultant feelings of failure. There is a need to maintain order, to be neat and be on time. Physically there is an irritation of the nerves, spinal column, and mucous membranes, as well as gastrointestinal problems.

Lettitia was given *Staphysagria,* from the *Staphisagria macrosperma* plant for her sensations of powerlessness, worthlessness, shame, and the suppressed anger that went along with those feelings. (Letitia said she wasn't angry and yet she admitted to chasing her half-sister around the house with a knife.) She was afraid to express her anger for fear of what would happen to her and to anyone upon whom she released her anger. The fears she experienced as a result of her abusive childhood and subsequent relationships led her to believe that speaking up was not an option. Her sexual abuse further decreased her sense of self and self-worth. Though seemingly confident externally, inside there was a deep sense of worthlessness. If I were to give the plant *Delphinium* to a well person in a toxic amount, I could replicate these feelings in that person even though they had not had the experiences that were part of Letitia's life.

Life's experiences for these superwomen culminated in varying dis-eases or expressions of energy—symptoms. When that energy, or the false self is no longer present, they are open to create greater health and vitality, to value who they are and participate in life from that perspective. Diane had to believe she could trust again and stop dwelling on past negative experiences visited upon her by her mother. Darlene's energy had to shift to knowing she did all she could do for her family and lift the guilt and grief from her spirit. Mary needed to experience calm, and know that things were not out of control anymore. She was not failing; she was surviving. Letitia needed to recognize she was worthy of having and speaking her opinion, and that she was neither worthless or powerless.

So, let's boldly declare:

I AM LOVED. I AM WELL. I AM GOD'S CHILD.

RESTORE

To bring back or re-establish.

Synonyms—return; implies a return to an original state after depletion or loss; to renew, a restoration of what had become faded or disintegrated so that it seems like new; repair; reconstruct; replace; strengthen; heal.

BALANCE

A situation in which different elements are equal or in correct proportion; an even distribution of weight enabling someone or something to remain upright and steady; good balance requires coordination of several parts of the body; similarly, balance requires coordination of the aspects and components of life.

Synonyms—bring back into line; equity—we do not all start from the same place and must acknowledge and make adjustments to imbalances; harmony—a state of peaceful existence and agreement.

CHAPTER 6

Where Do I Start?

Start where you are right now, today.

Nutrition

In *A Path to Healing* I have a chapter dedicated to nutrition where I include information on the detoxification diet, how to eat for better digestion and therefore elimination, and what to eat depending on your blood type. There are also sections on sugar, milk, and other substances that some people call food. Twenty-two years later there is more information I would like to share with you, because as I said earlier, learning requires repetition.

Before diving into those subjects, let me present some information about the "food" industry. The documentary "What the Health" offers insightful commentary on how organizations including the American Diabetes Association, the American Cancer Society, Susan G. Komen, and the American Heart Association influence the food industry. The purpose of the documentary is to expose the interconnectedness of some organizations and persuade people to become vegetarians. Though I do not believe that everyone should be a vegetarian, I do believe it important to understand the conflicts of interests that exist between these organizations and food manufacturers.

Companies like Dannon (maker of Dannon yogurt) and Kraft (makers of Velveeta, Oscar Mayer wieners, Lunchables) are corporate sponsors of the American Diabetes Association. The American Cancer

Society takes money from Tyson chicken, one of the biggest makers of processed chicken, and from Yum! Brands (Pizza Hut, KFC, Taco Bell).

Susan G. Komen, originally known as The Susan G. Komen Breast Cancer Foundation, partners with and receives money from KFC and Dietz & Watson, makers of processed meats. The American Heart Association takes hundreds of thousands of dollars from the beef industry (Texas Beef Council) and from poultry and dairy producers. It also takes in millions from fast food and processed food manufacturers.

In other words, all of these health organizations are taking money from companies that produce foodstuffs that are associated with the very diseases these organizations are supposedly fighting. The documentary makes the analogy that this would be like the American Lung Association taking money from the tobacco industry. And finally, the United States Department of Agriculture gets money from the meat and dairy industry, McDonald's, Hershey's and Dannon.

Perhaps you cannot afford all organic food and you must rely on the foods in commercial markets. Are you able to purchase one organic vegetable a week? Buy fresh kale or blueberries, things you do not peel as they are more susceptible to pesticides. Or buy a free-range chicken (no hormones, tranquilizers, or antibiotics) on occasion. What changes did our Superwomen make to benefit their health and save themselves?

Detoxification Diet

At the end of the first visit, I ask all my patients to record in a journal the foods they eat, how much water they drink, and their bowel habits for the next five days. This exercise is not only for my benefit, but also for theirs since I've found many people do not realize how much starch or sugar and how few vegetables and fruit they eat.

Superwoman Diane began her day with coffee, bagels and cream cheese, or a sugary cereal with whole milk. Lunch was often either non-existent or some fast-food option. Dinner was usually chicken and a salad or fries. Occasionally, she would have green beans or broccoli. She snacked on chips and salsa or cashews. She had maybe one eight-ounce glass of water a day and did not move her bowels regularly.

Darlene ate eggs and bacon or raisin bran cereal with whole milk for breakfast. A salad of iceberg lettuce, tomato, and tuna with onions and celery, along with crackers, was her lunchtime meal most days. Fried fish or chicken salad and a green vegetable was her dinner. Sometimes she had pizza. She too snacked on chips or dried cranberries. She drank three eight-ounce glasses of water in order to take her medication.

Mary's breakfast consisted of eggs and cheese with sausage and toast for three of the five days. She had oatmeal for two days. Lunch and, at times, dinner was a processed-meat ham or turkey sandwich complemented with either iceberg lettuce or soup and crackers. Once she had white rice, beans, and corn. Spinach was her only cooked green vegetable, which she had with fried fish, fried chicken, or baked salmon. She consumed six eight-ounce glasses of water each day, and had a small bowel movement daily.

Letitia's breakfast was oatmeal raisin cookies and garbanzo beans and sometimes Greek yogurt. Lunch was a sweet potato and vegetables. She snacked on peanuts and plantain chips. She ate chow mein noodles three times a week and moved her bowels every other day.

I asked my Superwomen/patients to do a 10-day detoxification diet which was primarily vegetarian. My patients do not have to eat everything on the "foods to include" list. However, when they eat, I ask if they will choose from the list. (For a comprehensive description of the detoxification diet please see pages 69-76 in *A Path to Healing: A Guide To Wellness for Body, Mind and Soul*). Fruits, vegetables (sautéed or steamed as well as salad), raw nuts, and seeds were a major part of the detoxification diet, as were beans and other high-fiber foods. I gave each woman a list of foods that have texture and color and flours that were multi-grain. These foods are necessary for cleansing the system and reducing the stress certain foods put on our bodies. Fish (only the fish that swim) was allowed for two or three meals when they'd decided they just could not eat one more carrot! White sugar and rice and flour were not recommended. Since preservatives and food additives were also forbidden, my Superwomen were tasked to read food labels to make sure to avoid them. Examples of common preservatives include sodium nitrite and sodium benzoate. Some common additives are high fructose corn syrup and food colorings. I asked them to eat organic to the best of their ability. Egg whites were fine, egg yolks were not. Cow's milk was also not part of the detoxification diet. Plant milks like almond, flax, rice, sprouted rice, coconut, and oat are welcomed. Also, during detox, I recommend exercising three times a week, even if it is only a 10-minute race walk.

There are supplements that I ask each patient to take as well. As I mentioned in the Stress chapter, I suggest borage oil, flax oil (both two capsules, one or two times a day) for anti-inflammatory and fiber effects, and liquid calcium/magnesium (one tablespoon before bed and one tablespoon any time of day). Very often when people are detoxifying from processed foods with preservatives, dyes, sugars, salts and fats, they can become agitated and irritable, and their sleep becomes disturbed. The liquid calcium/magnesium aids in calming the central nervous system.

Here is an example of the diet:

FOOD TO INCLUDE	FOODS TO AVOID
BEANS	
Black, red, pinto, kidney, black-eyed peas, chickpeas, split peas, lentils, lima beans. Aduki and mung beans are ideal for weight loss or weak digestive systems.	Canned (unless organic).

BEVERAGES	
Herb teas: mint, spearmint, comfrey, eucalyptus, dandelion, chaparral, red clover, chamomile. Celestial Seasonings teas. Coffee substitutes: Pero, Cafix, Roma, Yannoh.	Soft drinks, coffee, alcohol.
BREAD	
Millet, rye, buckwheat, 7-, 8-, or 21-grain. Soya tortillas, only whole grains, freshly ground free of all preservatives. Ezekiel 4:9 bread (freezer section of store).	White bread and blended made of enriched and white flour.
CEREALS/GRAINS	
Millet, oatmeal, brown and wild rice, barley, cornmeal, cracked wheat, 7 grain, quinoa, amaranth, spelt, buckwheat groats (freshly ground if possible), oatmeal, overnight oats.	Processed cereals which are puffed or flaked. No white rice/refined grains.
DAIRY PRODUCTS	
No dairy products. Tofu (soy cheese) is OK. Milk substitutes: soy, sesame or diluted tahini milk, rice milk, oat milk, almond milk, coconut milk. Use nut milks sparingly. Flax, sprouted brown rice, coconut, hemp.	Eggs in any form (except whites), milk, cheeses.

FATS	
Most cold-pressed, unsaturated oils such as: sesame and olive for medium to low heat, peanut, almond, safflower, and soy for high heat. Spectrum non-hydrogenated spread.	Butter, shortening, margarine, saturated oils, rancid and continually heated oils.
PROTEIN	
Tofu/ tempeh, seitan (unless gluten sensitivity), legumes. Meat subs: Boca Burgers (vegan original), Okra Courage Burgers (chicken), Tofurkey, Veggie Ground Round. Gimme Lean Light Life and St. Yves are popular brands. Mushrooms (portabella, shitake). Cold water fish such as salmon, halibut, mackerel, branzino, and sardines are allowed once or twice only if weakness occurs.	Beef, pork, chicken, turkey, seafood (shellfish; you can eat the fish that swim but not the fish that crawl).
SEASONING	
Chives, garlic, parsley, oregano, basil, marjoram, sage, thyme, cayenne, cumin, anise, fennel, ginger, and savory. Kelp, vegetable, and herb seasonings that contain no sodium chloride (table salt), including salt substitutes like Spike, Vegit, Veg Sal, Herbamare,	Spices, pepper, and table salt. White vinegar.

Bragg's Liquid Aminos. Dr. Bronner balanced mineral seasoning. Nutritional yeast. Unrefined sea salt. Pure apple cider, balsamic, or rice vinegar.	

VEGETABLES

Raw or freshly steamed, organically grown if possible. Artichokes, asparagus, beets, carrots, celery, chives, corn, cucumbers, endive, green beans, green peas, lentils, lima beans, onions, red peppers, green peppers, sweet potatoes, tomatoes, yams, watercress, kale, beet tops, radishes, red cabbage.	Sprayed, canned, or frozen vegetables.

SALADS

Buy organic. Fresh spring mix and vegetables, arugula, dandelion, radicchio, beet greens, romaine and bitter lettuce, spinach, tomatoes, cucumbers, green peppers. Dressings including Annie's, Newman's Own, and other healthy dressings without dairy, sugar, or white vinegar.	Sulphured and high sodium vegetables. Cheap salad bars. Iceberg lettuce.

DESSERTS	
Fresh whole fruits, fruit cocktails, fruit gelatin, whole tapioca. Sweeteners: Stevia, sorghum, Succanat, brown rice syrup, nonk fruit, Erythritol, and maple syrup (in moderation).	Candy, pastries, custards, sauces, and ice cream unless plant based. Sprayed and sulfured or canned or frozen fruit unless organic and frozen.
FRUITS	
Fresh fruits organically grown if possible. Apples, apricots, bananas, berries, cherries, currants, grapes, guavas, grapefruits, lemons, mangos, melons, nectarines, oranges, papayas, peaches, pineapples, pears, plums, persimmons, tangerines. Dried fruits (unsulphured).	
JUICES	
Only fresh UNSWEETENED juices if possible. Fruit: apple, berry, cherry, grape, grapefruit, lemon, orange, pear, pineapple, prune. Vegetables: beet, carrot, cucumber, celery, garlic, onion, peppers (red or green bell), radish, red cabbage, turnip, kale, collards. Peel sprayed vegetables or wash thoroughly. When juicing, **apples are the only fruit to combine with vegetables**.	All canned and frozen juices. Sweetened or blended juice. Juice from concentrate. Juice with added sugar.

NUTS & SEEDS	
Limited amounts of nuts, particularly fresh, raw (not roasted or salted): walnuts, almonds, and pecans. Nut butters: almond, Brazil and pine-nuts freshly made in the blender or juicer only. Seeds: sunflower, chia, sesame, and pumpkin.	Roasted and/or salted nuts and those high in fat such as cashews.
SOUPS	
Homemade soups made from vegetables. Brown rice, barley, lentils, or millet. Soup with vegetables.	Canned and creamed soups, bouillon, or dehydrated consommé.
POTATOES & PASTA & GRAINS	
Baked or steamed potatoes with jackets and mashed. All kinds of pastas made from whole grains such as durum semolina, millet, brown rice, buckwheat, and vegetable and bean flours without eggs. Baked sweet potatoes.	French fries, potato chips, grilled potatoes. Refined pasta, noodle, and macaroni products. **Avoid white potatoes, pastas, and other starchy vegetables for weight loss!**
SEA VEGETABLES	
Algae: agar, dulse, nori, wakame, kombu and kelp, hijiki and arame, Irish moss and corsican.	

SUGGESTED MENU		
Only a suggestion. You may eat dinner for breakfast (i. e, vegetables, beans, sweet potato).		
BREAKFAST	**LUNCH**	**DINNER**
Juice diluted with water Raw/cooked fruit Multi-grain ceral w/ plant milk Oatmeal or overnight oats in coconut milk or almond milk Rye or multigrain toast with a nut butter in moderation	Salad Soup Potato (sweet or blue) Steamed or sauteed vegetables Brown rice, quinoa, or millet and tofu/tempeh or beans	Steamed Vegetables Brown Rice Salad Beans Soup Potato
MID-MORNING	**MID AFTERNOON**	**EVENING**
Fresh fruit or juice diluted with a little water	Nuts or fruits	Diluted juice or fruit
You may desire to eat more frequently on this temporary diet. –Go right ahead!		

I also suggested that they have different eating habits to aid digestion and elimination. That is the purpose of the detox diet: to have better, more frequent, or larger eliminations. If we eat daily but do not defecate daily, we retain toxins in our system that create havoc with our immune system and organs. Imagine not emptying a garbage can. You would attract more flies and maggots, right? So, when you do not move your bowels regularly you are accumulating toxic waste that affects your organs. Constipation is one of the most common GI complaints. There can be many reasons for this inactivity of the bowels: not taking time to relax long enough to have healthy bowel habits, medications, not enough fiber in the diet, not enough exercise (the bowel is a muscle and it needs exercise as well), and of course, not enough water and other liquids.

I asked them to drink water 20 minutes before a meal and 45 minutes after a meal rather than with a meal, so as not to wash away the food and enzymes in the mouth. Digestion begins in the mouth, not in the stomach. I suggested they do not eat while watching TV, especially the news, as that produces a stress response and impairs digestion, as all the blood goes to the periphery of the body for fight or flight, and not to the core of the body for digestion. There is no good news. Nurturing oneself by eating silently, watching a comedy, or listening to some nice music is best for digestion and wellness.

I suggested to the best of their ability to please eat only organic foods. Especially the foods you cannot peel like kale, spinach, blueberries, grapes, and other fruits and vegetables. Why is that important? Organically grown fruits and vegetables have not been exposed to chemicals such as pesticides, fungicides, and fertilizers and are not genetically modified (where the genetic material has been artificially manipulated in a laboratory through bioengineering). The animal products do not contain tranquilizers (to keep them calm), antibiotics (to keep them dis-ease free because they are pinned up in such close quarters), or hormones (to get them fattened for slaughter sooner). Organic farming is also helpful for the environment, as it eliminates the chemical pollution of watersheds and soil. Moreover, organic foods have more nutrients— especially minerals—than foods produced commercially. It may be that you can only eat one organic vegetable a week. That is just fine. Do whatever you can. It also may be that you have a local farmer near you who may not be able to afford the certification for organic. Ask whether and what pesticides he or she uses. Perhaps the answer is none. Buy from them.

On her next visit, Diane reported she was feeling much better in every way. She said she felt emotionally lighter, happier, less moody, and that she was opening to people and reaching out to them. She said she was not thinking as much about all the negative circumstances she had with her mother or her divorce. She also felt physically lighter because she began moving her bowels daily. And her blood pressure numbers were moving back toward the normal range.

Because Darlene had diabetes, I allowed her to have fish once daily to support her blood sugar. But I also suggested she have the fish only with vegetables, not starches, in order to have a more complete digestion and elimination. I limited her fruits and increased her vegetable consumption. If she had fruit juice it had to be diluted and all natural. She told me she was not crying as much and didn't feel depressed anymore. She said she stopped thinking about the terrible things that had happened to her. She said she told herself those things are in the past. After our meeting she said she went home and noticed all the canned foods in her home and read the labels. She didn't want to waste it all, so she ate some of it then decided to donate the rest to a shelter.

Over time, her morning blood sugar level was closer to normal, not elevated as it had been in the past. She had increased her exercise from 10 minutes three times a week to four times a week. She had a day when she ate a fried chicken sandwich on white bread along with some chocolate and she immediately noticed how awful she felt. Though Darlene had been taking 17 medications, she eventually required only two. She proudly shared with me that she'd been doing well and told me, "I said hello to the new me."

Mary reported that she'd begun sleeping better as her anxiety and depression "really tapered off." She said she didn't get so upset about things anymore, her fears had decreased, and she was not feeling as out of control. Additionally, her pain was reduced after and she said she felt balanced and better. "I used to put me on hold. I don't do that anymore."

Letitia returned, reporting she too was feeling "really good in every way." She had lost five pounds and was not feeling as tired after working all day and on the weekends. She didn't have the aches and pains going up and down the steps (she had not told me about that). She was moving her bowels regularly, and said she was more relaxed and had more clarity. She also said there were things she had not shared with me, like she had been shot at by her ex-husband, had several abortions, and was homeless for a while. Her sleep was much better, as was her mood, and she told one of her children to figure out a situation she was having, rather than do it for her. She was spinning and doing yoga. She felt calm and well mentally and physically. She said she took the time to thank God for all that God was doing for her.

I typically repeat the homeopathic remedy at every session or, depending upon the concern, I may change it to match whatever energy the patient is expressing. It was now time to transition my super women to blood type diets.

Diets for Blood Types

White flour, sugar, and milk is not good for anyone. However, I first learned from Dr. James L. D'Adamo, my naturopathic physician, that real foods that were good for some people were not good for others. (Dr James L. D'Adamo, *One Man's Food Is Someone Else's Poison*. Health Thru Herbs, Inc, 1980 Toronto) (His son Dr. Peter D'Adamo. expanded his father's work in his book, *Eat Right 4 Your Type*, G.P. Putnam's Sons,1996 New York).

I had been a vegetarian for eight years when I met Dr. D'Adamo in 1978. I was tired all the time, had a face full of acne and was overweight by 30 pounds. Every year I'd get a cold and a sore throat. My blood type is B positive. Dr. D'Adamo told me I should not be vegetarian, and that animal protein was important for my body because of my blood type. That awareness changed my life, my career, and my health. Clinically, most of the information he taught me I have seen to be true in my practice, and I prescribe blood type diets for every patient.

After years of study in Europe, he observed that people needed different types of diets depending on their blood type. Understanding that all blood types can receive blood from blood type O's, it was thought that Blood type O's were the first blood type in our human evolution. Diane is blood type O. I explained to her that blood type O's were hunters and roamed their environment looking for animal protein for their nutrition. Ideally, people with this blood type have a highly energetic and active body. In an ideal world, an O should not be vegetarian and should consume animal protein like chicken, lamb, bison, fish (not shellfish) and turkey—all free range preferably. Starches and many beans are not something the O digests easily. Meat and vegetables are ideal unless there is some cancerous process. In that case I would have them be vegetarian for a time and then resume animal protein—only fish. They cannot get all their nutrients from foods and nutritional supplements are advised. Blood type O's are reliable and conscientious people/employees, being willing to take on the work of others and see it through to completion. They can tend to be very methodical and do not like to be rushed.

Blood type A's came into existence as we migrated out of Africa and mutated. These mutations included changes in facial structure and skin color for the ability to absorb more vitamin D. A's do not have high levels of hydrochloric acid that O's have, and thus do not digest meat as well. A's were people who didn't choose to continue to roam looking for animal protein, but rather built communities and cultivated crops. Their food requirements are of a lower vibration food, like the vegetable kingdom (a carrot has less energy than a cow or chicken). A's are very sensitive, and foods that do not agree with them can create rapid responses like headaches or acne. Being vegetarian is ideal for an A.

Mary's blood type is A. While my suggestion to patients to do a detoxification diet for 10 days is fairly sudden, I do not advise a sudden switch to being vegetarian in the long term. I asked Mary to stop red meats first, then chicken and poultry and then fish. This change may take six to eight months to accomplish. As I say to all my patients embarking on new habits, guilt is not an option. Do not beat yourself up if you have a piece of chocolate cake. Go to the next meal and do your best with each meal.

A's are the opposite of O's in that they have a low vibrational body and a very active nervous/mental system. They are busy. A's are more mental, O's more physical. Blood type A's always have a thought, plan, or project, so much so they cannot do it all. They have a lot of high nervous mental energy. Of course, all people can be impatient, and A's seem to be more impatient, and can therefore experience problems sleeping. Anxiety and worry are a big part of their lives.

Blood group B combines the best of both worlds–the intellect and empathy of blood group A and the need for physical activity of blood group O. Lettitia is a B and moderation is the key for a B, however. They need to be vegetarian three to four days a week and have animal protein (fish, turkey, lamb, rabbit) two or three days a week. The dietary requirements resemble both A and O. Like blood type O's, whole wheat is too acidic for B's, and corn, buckwheat, and peanuts can be problematic. To receive vegetable protein, beans are better for B's than tofu or tempeh. Unfortunately, chicken is not a food that a blood type B assimilates well. There is a type B agglutinating factor in the muscle tissue of the chicken that causes blood to clump, causing immune disorders and strokes. Fish is the animal protein source that works well for B's, especially, halibut, sole, sardines, flounder, cod, salmon, grouper, branzino, and monkfish.

It is thought that blood group B's had to be more flexible and creative in order to survive the intermingling of cultures of the O's and A's. There was not the need for the order of the A society and yet they also did not need to be nomadic and look for meat as the O once did. Type B's are more flexible and not so intense in their body or mind. Both mind and body are cultivated equally. They see other points of view and are empathetic, making good counselors, communicators, and motivators. Blood type B's could consider self-employment as they are self-starters and do not do well with management from/by others.

Finally, blood type AB, or the "universal recipient", came into existence. This is a rare blood type, as only about four to five percent of the population have this type. While they are a combination in personality type of A and B, they are not as sensitive as an A and have less nervous energy. High strung like an A and yet centered or easily gravitating to centering practices like a B, they are diplomatic and pleasant. Their foods are similar to an A and being vegetarian would be acceptable. However, they should have fish once or twice a month and do well with lamb, like a blood type B. Unlike a B, tofu is well tolerated by blood type AB's. Though Darlene is an AB, because she had high blood sugar, I suggested she have animal protein, especially fish, several times a week.

Find out your blood type and explore these suggestions. Perhaps it will assist in changing your life too.

Drink More Water

All of my Superwomen had to increase their water intake and I imagine you do as well. Water makes up almost 70 percent of our body composition. The body is approximately 60 percent water, the brain is approximately 70 percent water and the lungs are 90 percent water. Every cell, tissue, and organ has water in it. We need to drink one-half our body weight in ounces. If you are an athlete or breastfeeding, you will need more water (one liter per hour of exercise). For example, if you weigh 150 pounds you need to consume 75 ounces of fluid a day, mostly by drinking pure water.

We lose water daily in our perspiration, bowel, urine, and respiration (breath), and we must replace it. Lack of water causes dehydration, which reduces the amount of blood in your body and forces your heart to pump harder to deliver oxygen-bearing cells to your muscles. Thus, dehydration causes faster breathing and a faster heart rate. It also causes poor sleep since it blocks the production of melatonin,[46] a hormone from the brain which helps us sleep. Dehydration is connected to time of day (rising at night and decreasing in daytime), constipation, irritability (which can be from constipation), dizziness, headaches, poor memory and concentration, impaired judgment, fatigue (water aids in breaking down and transporting nutrients to use as energy), dry skin, decreased coordination, muscle weakness, yellow urine, and blood pressure changes, as your blood is thicker and blood flow therefore restricted.

If you are thirsty, you are already dehydrated.

What About Other Liquids in Place of Water?

It is true that you can get fluids through other sources such as herbal teas and foods that are 85 to 95 percent water like celery, cucumbers, oranges, and melons. Twenty percent of your fluid needs can come from foods composed of water. However, most of your fluid intake should be from pure water.

I am often asked about black tea, coffee, soft drinks, juices, and cocoa. You can make an argument for any liquid as a substitute for water but, like with prescription drugs, there can be unintended side effects. The caffeine in these liquids can be dehydrating for the body. Caffeine, found in four of the five liquids named above, acts as a mild diuretic in the body, causing more urination.[47] But more importantly, caffeine removes calcium from the bones and that can increase the risk of osteoporosis as we get older. And of course, we know coffee can produce anxiety, heart palpitations, digestive problems, heartburn, ulcers, constipation, diarrhea, and sleeplessness.

Decaffeinated coffee is not much better. Decaffeinated green tea would be a better option. Soft drinks can create the same effect and they also contain harmful sugar. Sodas are the leading cause of type 2 diabetes in this country, and diet sodas are even worse. They may contain aspartame, a substance that has methyl alcohol which, when entering the body, turns to formaldehyde. Formaldehyde is carcinogenic. When aspartame and carbohydrates are mixed, it causes your brain to slow the production of serotonin.[48] Serotonin is the hormone that allows you to feel happiness and balances your mood. Diet sodas also trigger the body to believe there is sugar in the blood and thus activate insulin from the pancreas. When there is no sugar to be found the body craves sugar. These substances also have purines (which cause a form of arthritis called gout) and other toxins. Most of the water in these substances is used to eliminate toxins out of the body. And the milk in cocoa milk is not really a drink. Cow's milk is for baby cows. The best source of fluids is still water.

What Does Water Do for Us?

Drinking water helps to lubricate the spinal cord and joints, as well as mucous membranes of our nose, mouth, and throat, it aids in digestion, and flushes toxins out of the body. If the toxins are not flushed, they get stored as fat cells. Water protects the brain by delivering glucose to it and keeps the body's temperature normal. If weight loss is your goal, drink the required amount of water, as it reduces your hunger. Without adequate water the organs wrinkle and weaken, like the largest organ, the skin. Collagen is affected by dehydration and that affects the firmness of the skin.

A 2016 study from the University of Illinois printed in *Journal of Human Nutrition and Dietetics* examined the dietary habits of more than 18,300 US adults. This study found that the majority of people who increased their consumption of plain water—tap water or from a cooler, drinking fountain or bottle–by one percent reduced their total daily calorie intake as well as their consumption of saturated fat, sugar, sodium and cholesterol. (An R, 2016)[49]

Water, or its lack (dehydration), can influence one's mental and emotional state. Mild levels of dehydration can produce disruptions in mood and our ability to reason and learn. This may be of special concern in the very young, very old, those in hot climates, and those engaging in vigorous exercise. Mild dehydration produces alterations in a number of important aspects of brain function such as concentration, alertness, and short-term memory in children (10 to 12 years old) (Bar-Or O, 1985)[50], young adults (18 to 25 years old) (D Anci KE, 2009)[51], and in the oldest adults (50 to 82 years old). (Suhr JA, 2004)[52] As with physical functioning, mild to moderate levels of dehydration can impair performance on tasks such as short-term memory, perceptual discrimination, arithmetic ability, visual-motor tracking, and psychomotor skills. (Cian C, 2001)[53]

Dehydration is a risk factor for delirium and for delirium presenting as dementia in the elderly and in the very ill. (Culp KR, 2004)[54] Recent work shows that dehydration is one of several predisposing factors in observed confusion in long-term care residents. (Voyer P, 2009)[55] Chronic dehydration can lead to fatigue, heartburn, arthritic pain, back pain, headaches, colitis pain, and leg pain. Good hydration is associated with a reduction in urinary tract infections, hypertension, fatal coronary heart disease, venous thrombo-embolism, and cerebral infarct. All of these effects need to be confirmed by clinical trials.

In 1995, Dr. F. Batmanghelidj wrote the book *Your Body's Many Cries for Water*. Reprinted in 2006, he writes, "Chronic cellular dehydration painfully kills. Its initial outward manifestations have until now been labeled as diseases of unknown origin." He further notes that "...water is a natural medicine for a variety of health conditions." (Batmanghelidj, 1992)[56]

Let's look at histamine. Allergies are caused by a histamine reaction in the body in the event of an allergic reaction, and hydration influences histamine levels. Histamine is involved in the inflammatory response, and it is our body's way of responding to foreign substances. It can be released in the nose or mouth, causing the tiny blood vessels to be more open to white blood cells (part of our immune system) that actually attack the foreign substances. This reaction causes fluid to move out of the tiny blood vessels and creates a runny nose and watery eyes. When the body becomes dehydrated, histamine levels rise to help preserve water in the body. Water regulates histamine.

It is a neurotransmitter that has two functions: immune support and water regulation. When your body is hydrated, histamine is barely noticeable. When you are dehydrated histamine is reacting. It is also triggered when your internal environment is acidic and dehydrated. It is produced to begin the process of water regulation when dehydrated. Many of us are acidic because of our SAD (Standard American Diet), which causes inflammation that in turn triggers histamine production. The acidity and the dehydrated body keep one in an irritated inflamed state.

I suggest the following to all my patients:
START EACH DAY WITH 2 TO 3 GLASSES (8 TO 10 OUNCES) OF WATER WITH SOME FRESH SQUEEZED LEMON OR LIME.

(If you are blood type A or AB, the water needs to be warm, and if you're blood type O or B, the water should be room temperature).

IN BETWEEN BREAKFAST AND LUNCH AND LUNCH AND DINNER DRINK 2 TO 3 MORE, DEPENDING ON YOUR WEIGHT. IF YOU HAVE ALREADY MADE THIS A HABIT, DRINK ONE MORE GLASS OF WATER A DAY THAN NORMAL.

Do this weekly until you achieve your desired goal. If it is winter, it is fine to drink warm water, but no sugar.

Reduce Sugar

Ketchup, barbeque sauce, soup, low fat yogurt, granola, fruit juice, sports drinks, spaghetti sauce, chocolate milk, coffee creamers, iced tea, protein bars, cereal bars, canned fruit, canned baked beans, breakfast cereals, premade smoothies, soft drinks, pastries, ice cream, candies, syrup—need I go on?—all contain sugar. And not the natural sugars. That is why I have been telling patients for years to read the labels.

What words are you looking for to let you know there is sugar in the product? Dextrose (produced from corn), maltodextrin, maltose, fructose, high fructose corn syrup, galactose, and sucrose. Be aware also that if any of these words are the first or second ingredient listed on a product label, there is a lot of sugar in the product.

Sugar is made from sugar cane or sugar beet stalks. It is cut down and sent to a factory to extract the cane juice. Molasses is present in sugar and it is removed with water and bone char – yes, the bones of animals, that are crushed and burned then mixed with water to take out the molasses and create the white crystals. Brown sugar contains slightly more molasses than refined sugar. According to PETA (People for the Ethical Treatment of Animals), the cattle bones are from Pakistan, India, Afghanistan, and Argentina. They are sold to traders in Scotland, Egypt, and Brazil who sell them to the US sugar industry. Turbinado sugar or "sugar in the raw" is only boiled once and so is less refined than white sugar and bone char is not used. However, both white sugar and Turbinado sugar have the same calories and carbs.

In animal studies, sugar has been found to produce more symptoms than is required to be considered an addictive substance. Animal data have shown significant overlap between the consumption of added sugars and drug-like effects, including binging, craving, tolerance, withdrawal, and opioid effects. Sugar addiction seems to be dependent on the natural endogenous opioids (hormones for pain relief, increased mood, and lessened anxiety) that get released upon sugar intake. In both animals and humans, the evidence in the literature shows substantial parallels and overlap between drugs of abuse and sugar, from the standpoint of brain neurochemistry (brain hormones) as well as behavior. (DiNicolantonio JJ, 2018)[57]

One of the most important brain hormones is serotonin. It is made from tryptophan, an amino acid, and is needed for mood stabilization and happiness. Tryptophan is found in eggs, cheese, tofu, salmon, nuts and seeds, turkey, and pineapples. Exercise, positive thoughts, high fiber diets to increase gut bacteria, and sunshine also increase your levels of serotonin.

Beta-endorphins, another type of brain hormone, are released from the pituitary gland in the brain during stress and exercise. They act on the opiate receptors in the brain, promoting pleasure and reducing pain. They are also the reason why we crave comfort foods. Fatty, sugary, highly processed foods like cakes and pies, macaroni and cheese, potatoes and French fries all raise our blood sugar rapidly and the beta-endorphins follow. As with serotonin, exercise, meditation, and sunshine also increase beta-endorphins. Herbs and foods including ginseng, oranges, grapes, strawberries, and chocolate (preferably 85 percent or higher cacao, vegan, low sugar, and with no artificial flavors or preservatives) are also a great option.

Randomized clinical trials and epidemiologic studies have shown that people who consume added amounts of sugar, especially sugar-sweetened beverages, tend to gain more weight, be obese, and have type 2 diabetes mellitus. In addition, they have increased triglycerides and cholesterol that lead to clogged arteries, cardiovascular issues, and hypertension. Basically, sugar leads to cellular inflammation and chronic degenerative disease.

Added sugars include all sugars used in processed or prepared foods, such as sugar-sweetened beverages, fruit drinks, dairy desserts, candy, ready-to-eat sugary processed cereals, white flour yeast breads, and white rice that turns to sugar in the body. (Quanhe Yang, Zefeng Zhang, Edward W. Gregg, & al, 2014)[58] While no form of sugar is good for you, there are sugars that are less harmful such as stevia leaf extract, sucanat, erythritol and monk fruit. You may be wondering why I didn't mention agave nectar. Agave nectar is primarily fructose. While fructose doesn't affect blood sugar significantly, regular consumption may increase cholesterol and triglycerides, as well as increased risk of fatty liver disease and insulin resistance. (Weber KS, 2018)[59] (Dornas WC, 2019)[60]

Stevia comes from a plant called *Stevia rebaudiana* and has been used for hundreds of years. It is sold as a highly concentrated liquid or in packets. Being much sweeter than table sugar, you only need a small amount. Always get the ninety-five to one hundred percent stevia extract, or there may be fillers and sugar alcohols in the product.

The best thing about stevia is that it is carbohydrate- and calorie-free. Studies have shown that stevia does not increase blood sugar levels as does sugar or other artificial sweeteners. Adults who ate a 290-calorie snack made with stevia, ate the same amount of food at the next meal as those who ate a 500-calorie snack made with sugar. They also reported similar fullness and satisfaction levels, although stevia does have an aftertaste. Animal studies show an improved sensitivity to insulin, the hormone that lowers blood sugar, and the release of some appetite suppressing hormones. Other studies have linked stevia consumption to decreased triglycerides, which are not so good fats, and increased HDL (good cholesterol) levels, creating a lesser risk of heart disease.

Sucanat is a natural cane sugar that is also made by extracting the juice from the sugar cane. It is less processed and needs no chemicals or bone char to get it from a plant to consumption. Unlike granulated sugar, which is composed of sucrose, sucanat is made up of sucrose, glucose, and fructose. It retains some molasses (which you'll recall comes from refining sugar cane or sugar beets) and has trace nutrients like iron, calcium, potassium, and vitamin B. It is still sugar and therefore can affect your blood sugar.

Erythritol is relatively new even though it was discovered in the 1800s. It wasn't until the 1990s that Japan began to use it in their foods.[61] Erythritol is made by fermenting the sweet, natural starches in fruits like pears and melons. Basically, good bacteria eat the starch and turn it into erythritol. It's like the fermentation process of yogurt, wine, and beer. It does not taste as sweet as sugar, and it also doesn't cause an increase in insulin levels. Erythritol is not absorbed into your digestive system like sorbitol or xylitol, which can cause digestive problems. Some of it is a chemical compound made from the fermentation of corn. However, in one study, high levels of erythritol have been shown to be associated with cardiovascular events.[62] As with all sugar, use sparingly.

Monk fruit is much sweeter than table sugar, has no calories or carbohydrates, and does not raise blood sugar. To date, it has no known side effects. The sweetener is derived from the dried fruit, which is a small melon native to southern China. It has been used in Traditional Chinese Medicine[63] for decades as an anti-inflammatory agent, to reduce sore throats and upper respiratory congestion, and to keep blood sugars stable. More research is needed, however, to determine its effectiveness.

WHATEVER YOU DO, AVOID ASPARTAME, SUCRALOSE, AND SACCHARIN. USE ALL SUGAR IN MODERATION.

Do Not Drink or Eat Dairy

Every one of my patients will say that for years I have been telling them milk is for baby cows, not humans. Not only are we the only animal that drinks milk as adults, but we are also the only animal that drinks milk from another animal. You will never see a giraffe go to a kangaroo, or a rabbit go to a mouse for milk. Even cows do not go back to their mothers after their four stomachs are formed. They eat plants! It would be like breastfeeding at age five. Dairy products include yogurt, Lactaid, cow's cheese, and butter.

"We could be putting gorilla milk on our cereal or having zebra milk and cookies. Why cow's milk? Using the animal that produces the largest quantity of milk but is more easily housed than an elephant means more money for the farmers," say the authors of *Skinny Bitch*, Rory Freedman and Kim Barnouin. (Freedman, 2005)[64] It's all about the money needed for advertising and packaging. The dairy industry is a multibillion-dollar industry.

So, what's wrong with cow's milk? I'm glad you asked. Milk and other dairy products are the top sources of saturated fat that clogs arteries. Milk also contains saturated fat. Diets high in saturated fat and cholesterol increase the risk of heart disease, type 1 and type 2 diabetes, and Alzheimer's disease. Studies also have linked dairy to an increased risk of breast, ovarian, and prostate cancer. (Aune D, 2015)[65] (DiNicolantonio JJ, 2018)[66] (Knut Dahl-Jørgensen, 1991)[67] And countries that consume more dairy have higher rates of multiple sclerosis. (Malosse D, 1992)[68]

We need the enzyme lactase to digest the lactose, or sugar, in milk. Between the ages of 18 months and four years, we lose the majority of that enzyme. Most of the world's population cannot digest cow's milk because of a lactose intolerance, and milk is the most common self-reported food allergen in the world. (Rona RJ, 2007)[69] When the undigested sugar mixes with cow's milk, it creates a growth of bacteria in the intestines that causes an acidic environment and subsequent inflammation[70]—and even cancer. Flatulence, gas, bloating, cramps, and diarrhea can follow. Another pro-inflammatory property of milk is D-galactose, a breakdown product of lactose. Pasteurization destroys enzymes that help break down proteins, diminishes vitamin content, and denatures the proteins in milk. Undigested milk proteins in the small intestine can damage the lining of the gut, cause inflammation, and affect the body's ability to absorb nutrients.

You may have seen A2 milk. What is A2 milk? Another way to get you to buy milk. There is some evidence that a proportion of people have an inability to digest casein, a protein found in dairy. This protein is divided into 2 types, A1 and A2. Only cow's milk in the western world contains A1, due to evolution of the protein, as cows were bred to be larger and produce more milk. All other milk including human, goat, and sheep's milk contains A2 protein which is easier to digest. The A2 milk company says their milk is easier to digest. Unfortunately, the symptoms of lactose intolerance and removing A1 from milk are very similar.

As mentioned, cow's dairy can increase the production of acid in the stomach. This results in a weakening of the bones. A study in Sweden found that women consuming more than three glasses of milk a day had almost twice the mortality (more than twenty years) compared to those women consuming less than one glass a day. And those who drank more milk did not have improved bone health; rather, they had more fractures—particularly, hip fractures.[71]

In contrast, people living on continents like Africa and Asia who do not drink much milk have decreased rates of osteoporosis. African women do not suffer from the same rates of osteoporosis as American women. Of the forty tribes in Tanzania and Kenya, only one tribe suffers with osteoporosis–the Masai. The Masai own cattle and drink milk. Higher dairy intake has also been linked to increased risk of prostate cancer.[72]

Milk intake has been implicated in acne, ear infections, frequent colds, and constipation.[73] In my practice, when I've encountered children who have frequent colds or eczema, I take them off of milk immediately. That action alone reduces the number of colds and eczema. The homeopathic remedy and herbs I prescribe complete the job of restoring the child to good health.

"Dairy products produce mucus." There are arguments and studies for and against this statement. It depends on who is funding the study as to what results are published. I encourage you to test yourself. Stop drinking milk for ten days; then start drinking it again for ten days. You decide if it's good for you.

Eat some tofu, tempeh almonds, leafy greens (kale, collards, mustards, bok choy), okra, kelp, seaweed, broccoli, beans, and nut milks to get calcium. And for your vitamin D needs, eat more mushrooms, wild caught mackerel, herring, salmon, sardines and tuna, eggs in moderation, and get some sunshine.

Finally, during the winter, all of my patients are taking Vitamin D3 2,000 to 5,000 iu's a day depending on their levels, zinc 25 to 35 mg a day, vitamin C 1,000 to 3,000 mg a day and for some, Quercetin 500 mg a day.

You're well on your way, so affirm for yourself:
I AM LOVED. I AM WELL. I AM GOD'S CHILD.

CHAPTER 7

Go to Sleep (What a Concept)

Sleep deprivation is not new. For the past 14 to 15 years, sleep deprivation has been a growing problem. Studies by the Centers for Disease Control and Prevention reported in their Morbidity and Mortality Weekly Report, their National Health Interview Survey 2020 69:504, that the number of Americans who sleep less than six hours per night increased from 28 percent to almost 33 percent over the last 15 years.

The pandemic made it worse. According to the American Academy of Sleep Medicine in their Sleep Prioritization Survey 2021, on Sleep Aid Use, 56 percent of the 2,000 people interviewed had sleep problems during the pandemic. I would echo that for the patients in my practice. Perhaps even more of them commented on sleeping poorly due to grief, anxiety, anger, and feelings of isolation and loneliness. "Sleep problems" range from taking up to an hour to fall asleep, waking in the middle of the night and not being able to get back to sleep, to not sleeping at all on some nights, but rather constantly tossing and turning through the night. Now that we are returning to a more "normal" way of life, it is a bit better.

However, whether I ask the question "How much water do you drink?" or "How much sleep do you get?" the answer is the same. "Not as much as I should." Repeatedly, my new patients tell me they are fatigued and *may* get five to six hours of sleep per night. Many go on to tell me that they have the TV on a timer, so it turns off once they're asleep. Or they report reading, working in bed, looking at their phones, playing a video game, or checking the internet until their eyelids meet.

Your bedroom is not your office, family room or den. And if it does function as all three, you've got to create some boundaries. Your bedroom is where you go to rest, sleep, and be rejuvenated. I counsel my patients to remove the TV from the bedroom and put phones, laptops, I-pads, and all electronics in another room at least one hour before getting into bed. Mental activity may increase stress hormones before bed.[74] And the blue light from your devices blocks melatonin, the hormone needed to make us sleepy. You can install a blue light blocker or get a pair of blue light blocking glasses if it's imperative for you to use your devices before bed.[75]

For some of you Superwomen, there may not be enough time to sleep for 7 to 8 hours every night. I understand. I ask that you give yourself two nights a week to get 7 to 8 hours sleep. I ask that you make it a priority for yourself and ultimately for your family. If your partner (male or female) or your children's biological father is participating, great. If not, is there a grandmother, sister, brother, godmother, great aunt, cousin, friend, or co-worker who could give you a gift of watching one or two of your children overnight? You will not receive a yes if you do not ask. If you have an infant or toddler, ask any or all of the people listed above to come in your home and assist you occasionally. Also know that this too shall pass.

Generally, people need seven to nine hours of sleep. I know I am one of those people. When we do not get enough sleep we eat more, typically of the wrong thing, thinking our body wants food for energy. However, what it really wants is sleep. Weight loss is more difficult when you do not get enough sleep every night.[76]

Of course, our moods and attitudes are also challenged and less than pleasant when we do not get enough sleep. Thinking and mental tasks are more difficult and our energy is low. I know when I do not get enough sleep (like when I was writing this book in addition to being in my practice most days of the week), I feel dull, sluggish, and less than enthusiastic about the day. I'm less patient, out of balance and not as crisp, clear, or sharp in my thinking. Do you notice that these bodily changes are like being dehydrated? The pillars of good health for me are nutrition, which includes drinking adequate amounts of water, regular exercise, physical and spiritual, and adequate amounts of sleep.

Sleep boosts short-term and long-term reasoning, problem solving ability, and intellect. Our genes that control our circadian rhythms (the built-in process that regulates sleep, hunger, and energy; our body clock) are affected by lack of sleep, so that our brains have a difficult time performing tasks like concentrating and learning new things. (I will talk more about the body clock on the next page, along with the different phases of sleep). Coordination and reaction time may be delayed or decreased, making you at higher risk for accidents in or out of your home. During sleep, pathways form between nerve cells, called neurons, in the brain to assist us in learning and remembering new things. Lack of sleep reduces the activity in the hippocampus, which is the memory center of your brain.[77] Sleep promotes the removal of waste products and toxins from the brain. And insomnia is a risk factor for developing or recurring depression.

Your immune system is weakened when you do not have enough sleep. During sleep your immune system produces infection-fighting substances like antibodies. Their job is to protect you from bacteria and viruses. Your body needs sleep to fight infectious diseases. Lack of sleep also creates a longer recovery time if/when you do become ill.

Lack of sleep creates greater fluctuations in blood sugar and makes diabetes harder to manage.[78] Too little sleep can increase insulin resistance. Sleep loss also has other health consequences such as hypertension, obesity, depression, heart attack, and stroke. The body needs an opportunity to rest and sleep in order to manage the stress and stress reactions of the day and of life.

I ask all my patients to go to bed the day before they wake up. So, go to bed before midnight and wake up the next day preferably after seven to eight hours of sleeping. All too often patients tell me they do get seven hours of sleep. It's just that those seven hours are from one in the morning to eight in the morning. Let's look at why this is not ideal.

There are four stages of sleep. Our brain activity begins to slow down, indicating phase one and then phase two of light sleep. This is followed, hopefully, by deep stage three and four sleep. This phase is the most difficult from which to awaken. It may not be the eight hours of sleep that people say makes them tired, but rather, at which part of the cycle they awaken. Without deep sleep we have a higher risk of cardio-vascular disease, diabetes, obesity, and stroke.[79] Deep sleep promotes growth hormones, immunity, bone and muscle repair and growth, and counteracts aging. The brain processes what we learned during the day.

REM sleep begins next after ninety minutes of sleep, as we sleep in ninety-minute cycles of non-REM (rapid eye movement) and REM. Non-REM (stage three and four) is deeper and more restorative.

The bulk of deep sleep should be the first one to four hours of sleep, and the final half of sleep should have the longest REM sleep, but no more than 25 percent of total sleep time or two hours. There are also more non-REM cycles in the beginning of the night. As the sun rises there is more REM sleep. This is when dreams are more readily available. Regardless of when you go to bed, the shift from non-REM to REM sleep happens at certain times. So, going to bed after midnight means you are losing that part of sleep that is most beneficial. This is clearly a problem for night shift workers and bartenders. Shift work has been linked to heart disease, obesity, and cognitive issues.

There is an area in the brain called the circadian timer which matches the movement and function of cells to the levels of light and darkness with the rotation of the earth every twenty-four hours. All life forms have a circadian rhythm. Several chemicals are released within a daily cycle that support the sleep/wake cycle (a circadian rhythm of sleep and wakefulness). This cycle influences brain wave activity patterns, cell repair, and hormone levels. For example, serotonin is made as soon as your eye perceives light and tells your body it is time to wake up. Serotonin stimulates your brain waves.

Adenosine is a drowsiness compound that builds up in the brain during the daytime. As darkness comes there are messages sent through the eyes to the pineal gland, and serotonin is turned into melatonin, using the essential amino acid, L-tryptophan. Melatonin is a hormone released by the pineal gland in the evening telling us it is time to sleep. Its production is highest between two and four o'clock in the morning. The higher the stress hormones of adrenal cortisol in the body, the lower the amounts of melatonin.

Affected by light, temperature, and food, the sleep-wake cycle helps keep us on a 24-hour schedule. So, bright lights at night such as our televisions and devices create wakefulness. The circadian rhythm, or internal clock, keeps the body in sync with the sun. This body clock controls not only waking and sleeping, but also body temperature (lowest before dawn), blood pressure regulation (highest in the evening), alertness (highest in mid-morning and early evening), intestinal activity (peaks in the morning), and hormone production. The 90 minutes before midnight is the time the body is most replenished, and cells are restored. It is also the best time to bring the adrenaline levels down. Adrenaline is the hormone responsible for the fight or flight reaction when you are stressed. (Sleep, 2020)[80]

Believe it or not, your genetic makeup dictates whether you're more comfortable going to bed earlier or later within that rough eight-to-midnight window, says Dr. Allison Siebern, an insomnia and sleep expert and professor in the Stanford University School of Medicine. "That means night owls shouldn't try to force themselves to bed at nine or ten if they're not tired. Of course, your work schedule or family life may dictate when you have to get up in the morning. But if you can find a way to match your sleep schedule to your biology—and get a full eight hours of Z's—you'll be better off," she said. So, go to bed. I tell my patients to just go to bed around 10 or 11 o'clock two nights a week to start and see what happens.

Ask yourself if you sleep well. Do you fall asleep within 10 to 15 minutes of getting in the bed? Do you wake up frequently, once, or not at all? If you wake up, which many of us do, do you fall back to sleep easily? And most importantly, do you wake up feeling rested, alert, and focused? If not, there are habits, supplements and herbs you may want to incorporate into your sleep habits.

I suggest to my patients, ideally:

- Have a routine (turn off all devices an hour before bed, take a hot shower and, as the body temperature drops, you should become drowsy) and a schedule.
- Go to bed at the same time.
- Wake up at the same time.
- Write down on a piece of paper all the things—ideas, worries, thoughts—that you believe will keep you from sleeping and tear it up. In other words, empty your mind.
- Write down on a separate piece of paper the things you need to do the next day, if you have not already put them in your phone calendar.
- No alcohol, coffee, caffeinated tea, or food before bed.
- If you must eat, eat protein not carbohydrates (breads, potatoes, and pastas).
- Do not drink anything before bed or more than 2 to 3 hours after dinner.
- Playing instrumental sleep music before getting into bed is fine.
- Use white or pink noise if you have to listen to something.
- Avoid excessive exercise before bed (stretching and yoga are okay); during the day, aerobic and weight training exercise or the use of resistance bands is great.
- Use an eye mask and ear plugs (the kind for swimmers) if you are sensitive to light and noise.
- Stimulate an acupuncture point behind and below the ear with your finger.
- Set the temperature at 65 to 68 degrees Fahrenheit (or

whatever is cool to you), as this makes for a better nights' sleep. (Heat exposure affects wakefulness and decreases slow wave sleep and REM sleep. Cold exposure may affect the heart, however. Thus, a cool temperature is best).
- Make sure you do not set the alarm to go off during a deep sleep phase; complete the cycle if you can. (Cutting the cycle short makes one feel worse on waking; cutting into a light sleep phase is better).
- Get sunlight throughout the day, especially in the morning (this helps to regulate our inner clock and differentiate between day and night).
- Go for a short morning walk to get sunlight and exercise.
- Do not nap longer than 30 minutes and do this earlier in the day.
- Meditate before bed.
- Tighten and relax every muscle, including facial muscles.

You may also want to use some botanical (herbal) preparations for sleep. In my practice I suggest *Valeriana officinalis* (valerian), *Matricaria chamomilla* (German chamomile), or *Chamaemelum nobile* or *Anthemis nobilis* (Roman chamomile), *Passiflora incarnata* (purple passionflower), and *Lavandula angustifolia* (English lavender). I make a tincture (an herbal preparation of the herbal extract soaked in alcohol for a few weeks/months) of valerian, chamomile, and passiflora combined, and ask patients to take 30 drops in a little warm water ½ hour before bedtime.

Valerian has been used for centuries to calm the brain and central nervous system. There are substances in valerian that acts on GABA receptors. GABA (gamma aminobutyric acid) is a chemical messenger that helps to regulate impulses in the nervous system. It is one of the main neurotransmitters responsible for sleep and creates a sedative effect in the body. I use valerian as an anti-anxiety preparation as well.

The Egyptians used chamomile for fevers and shivering, as

a uterine tonic to increase blood flow, as an anti-inflammatory agent, especially for the skin, and as a sedative. I use it primarily as a sedative, and as a soap or lotion for irritated skin, mild eczema, and acne. Patients find the tea before bed to be very soothing and relaxing. Combined with ginger, chamomile is very useful in soothing stomach upset that creates gas, indigestion, and diarrhea. Homeopathically, chamomile is one of the remedies used for very irritable, defiant children, and for teething babies and toddlers.

Passiflora is historically used for diarrhea, nerve pain, hysteria, sleeplessness, and pain during menstruation. Today this herb is continuing to be useful for those circumstances, as well as for anxiety. Like valerian, it is thought to increase levels of GABA in the brain, which lowers the activity of some brain cells and makes you feel more relaxed.

Lavender may be used as a soap, essential oil, a spray for your pillow, incense, or all the above. It is primarily grown in parts of France, Italy, England, and Croatia. Many years ago, it was used as an herb for food and to comfort the stomach. Now it is mainly used as a nervine and in the essential oil form, assisting with anxiety.

Another herb that is useful, especially when mixed with the mineral magnesium, is ashwagandha. Native to Africa and India, it has been used for centuries in Ayurvedic medicine. It is an adaptogen which means it helps the body adjust to internal and environmental stressors. It helps to produce hormones like GABA and serotonin. With its calming effect and its ability to reduce cortisol, it is useful for restlessness, poor concentration, sleep disturbances, and anxiety.

Magnesium is a mineral that calms the central nervous system and is a key mineral for many enzymes, as well as muscle and nerve function. Chronically low levels can increase the risk of high blood pressure, heart disease, type 2 diabetes, and osteoporosis. It is useful in combatting stress, maintaining cardiovascular health, and supporting the immune system. The best way to get magnesium is through green leafy vegetables, beans, whole grains, nuts, and seeds. Low levels of magnesium correlate with poor sleep quality and insomnia. The Sleep Foundation says research shows that magnesium helps people to fall asleep faster and reduces early morning waking. In addition to eating plenty of leafy greens, nuts, and seeds (especially flax) I advise most of my patients to take magnesium (150 to 300 mg) before bed every night. It improves the hours you are asleep in the bed and not just the hours you are in the bed trying to sleep. A hot bath with epsom salts, which are made with magnesium, may also be useful as the body absorbs the salts through the skin.

DO NOT TAKE ANY OF THE HERBS OR MINERALS WITHOUT CONSULTING A NATUROPATHIC PHYSICAN. IF YOU DO, DISCONTINUE AFTER 3 MONTHS IF YOU DO NOT RECEIVE THE DESIRED EFFECT.

SLEEP WELL.

And don't forget to affirm for yourself:

I AM LOVED.   I AM WELL.   I AM GOD'S CHILD.

CHAPTER 8

Exercise (Baby Steps are Fine)

Since I have been talking to you, I see the benefits of exercise; my blood sugar is even better.

– Darlene

Exercise just makes you feel and sleep better.

– Diane

I'm race walking three times a week and I am sleeping good.

– Mary

I have to exercise now or I do not feel as well; it's amazing.

– Letitia

"Just Do It" – Nike

Whether it is going up and down your stairs 10 times a day (not to do laundry, just to exercise), following a YouTube video, jumping rope, jumping jacks, race walking outside, hiking, marching in place inside, calisthenics, squats, lunges, burpees, dancing or chair dancing to your favorite music by yourself, swimming, hula hooping, yoga, pilates, or a regimented boot camp, JUST DO IT!

Why? How many reasons do you need? Here are a few:

- Boosts the immune system by affecting white blood cells that eliminate bacteria and viruses from the body
- Increases blood flow, and circulation, thus helping to reduce blood pressure
- Reduces stress hormones (adrenaline, which increases your heart rate and blood pressure and cortisol, which increase sugars in the bloodstream—the "fight or flight" hormones) and therefore inflammation
- Increases the body's endorphin levels which are responsible for mood elevation and reducing pain
- Alleviates depression and anxiety
- Increases the level of high-density lipoproteins (the good cholesterol) and decreases the low-density lipoproteins (the bad cholesterol)
- Helps to decrease total cholesterol and triglycerides
- Improves cardiac/heart function, deterring heart disease, by increasing contractility of heart chambers
- Lowers resting heart rate, and strengthens the heart
- Increases metabolism, or the number of calories you burn a day, which leads to weight loss
- Decreases appetite when you exercise from 20 minute to one hour
- Along with the appropriate food, decreases blood sugar and A1C hemoglobin (the measurement of your blood sugar over a three-month period of time), and boosts your body's sensitivity to insulin
- Insulin sensitivity is increased, and your muscle cells can use any available insulin to take up the sugar in your body during exercise and after exercise
- Strengthens bones while toning and firming muscle
- Increases quality of sleep
- Increases self-confidence and self-esteem when clothes look and feel better

- Improves concentration and emotional stability
- Stimulates a feeling of well-being and accomplishment
- Improves brain health and reduces your chances of cognitive decline
- Boosts memory, decision making, problem solving, and attention
- Reduces overall the risk of dis-ease
- Improves balance and lowers risk of falling
- Increases endorphins, the brain's feel-good substances

Exercise is a main activity for detoxifying because you are using your lungs by exchanging carbon dioxide for oxygen, using the skin by sweating, and if you are drinking more water, you are enabling the bladder and the bowels to eliminate more efficiently.

I have learned to ask patients to start with 10 minutes three times a week. When I have asked for more, they will say they did not have 20 minutes, for example, so they did nothing. If you have more than 10 minutes or can do 10 minutes daily, please do so. Start slowly and work up to a race walk if you have not exercised before or are obese. Baby steps are important. You are not preparing for a marathon. And I do want you to set yourself up to win and succeed at whatever goal you set for yourself. At some point I'd like sweating to be a goal.

Once you have taken the baby steps of 10 minutes three times a week, the duration of your aerobic exercise could be 15 to 60 minutes. A common duration is 30 minutes. And the frequency on average could be three times a week, with no more than 48 hours between workouts. If you have not exercised in years, progress slowly.

It's best if your exercise has a warmup period of five to 10 minutes, which includes stretching, calisthenics, or the intended activity done slowly. If you break out into a light sweat, that is appropriate. Then continue with 15 to 60 minutes of whatever activity you choose and five to 10 minutes of cool-down, slowing down the activity, and stretching again. By the end of the cool-down, your heart rate should be under

100 beats per minute. If time permits, rest a bit after the exercise.

It is thought that regular exercise, in addition to other lifestyle changes and behaviors, protects against an initial cardiac event, aids in recovery after an event, and helps reduce the risk of recurring cardiac events.

For strength training you may choose to do three to five days a week, alternating between upper and lower body muscles, allowing at least 24 hours in between workouts of the same muscle group. The intensity could be such that you can only perform five to 15 repetitions. Like with aerobic exercise, there should be a warmup of stretching and performing a few repetitions with 50 percent of the intended weight of the actual exercise. Once you start the lifting, it is suggested to lift for two seconds, pause, and then lower for four seconds. Exhale as the weight is lifted and inhale as the weight is lowered.

According to Adele Diamond, in "Effects of Physical Exercise on Executive Functions: Going Beyond Simply Moving to Moving with Thought," published in the *Annals of Sports Medicine and Research* 2.1 (2015), strength training increases executive functions. Examples of executive functions are thinking before you act, exhibiting inhibitory control, thinking outside the box or having an "aha" moment, an awareness that seems to come out of nowhere, and being able to hold on to information.

IF YOU HAVE CARDIOVASCULAR, DIABETIC, OR PULMONARY CONCERNS, HAVE AN ASSESSMENT BEFORE ENGAGING IN STRENUOUS EXERCISE. YOUR EXERCISE PRESCRIPTION NEEDS TO BE INDIVIDUALIZED.

The past couple of years I have been grieving the death of my mother who lived to be 100 years old. I can tell you, aside from grief counseling, nothing has assisted me more than physical and spiritual exercises to get through the day.

In my 35 years of practice, I have found people with blood type O need physical activity not only for their bodies, but their memory and concentration as well. While exercise may not be what they want to do, it is an absolute necessity for better health. Perhaps more than any other blood type, aerobic exercise is one of the best treatments for blood type O's. They are generally muscular and brawny and require intense, frequent exercise to stimulate themselves and their minds. Jogging, spinning, and boot camps are all activities that would benefit an O blood type. Without this exercise there is a tendency to laziness and lethargy. Exercise is also important because it helps the body release toxins from the uric acid build-up from animal protein that they also must have as part of their diet.

As I said earlier, people with blood type A are different. They function on mental nervous energy and therefore jogging and boot camps (except for weight loss) are not recommended as those activities will excite and exhaust the A. Swimming, cycling, and race walking are great aerobic exercises for an A. And for the mind, the softer, gentler martial arts like tai chi, aikido, and qigong (chi gung) help calm the central nervous system and are easy on the joints. While I recommend yoga and meditation for almost everyone, A's benefit greatly from practices that calm the mind.

A person with blood type B has exercise needs that are shared with O and A. There should be some intense exercise three times a week for the physical body of a B, and yet their mind and nervous system also needs the calming effects of yoga and meditation.

People with AB blood type are stronger in personality and stamina than an A, and are able to tolerate moderate exercise like cycling without the nervous system being taxed. They also need calming exercises like yoga, aikido, and tai-chi. Meditation is also highly recommended.

Do some exercise you love and do it often. Do different exercises. Set goals that you know you can achieve. Maintain a schedule and know this is *your* time for *your* self-love and self-care. *You know what to say!*

I AM LOVED. I AM WELL. I AM GOD'S CHILD.

CHAPTER 9

Listening to What's Within/ Meditation/Spiritual Exercises

*Meditation brings me into a oneness I cannot explain;
it quiets the universe, brings comfort, focus and trust.
It's centering.*

–Diane

*One significant thing you encouraged is meditation;
I had worrying thoughts and now they are gone.*

–Darlene

*Meditation brings a calmness; a letting go of the noises from the day
and I hear my inner voice.*

–Letitia

A Way to Begin

When I sit down to meditate, this is what happens. I say the word "Ani-HU" and then a thought appears. *I have to go to the store.* Again I say, "Ani-HU" (said silently breathing out). And another thought. *Call Walter.*

"Ani-HU" (breathing out). *Remember to send the vitamin D to Ms. Smith.* "Ani-HU" (breathing out) *Make the dinner reservation for Sean's birthday.* "Ani-HU" (breathing out).

After about five to 10 minutes, I am focused on my breathing and the word "Ani-HU" (I pronounce it "an-eye-hue"—I will explain the meaning shortly), and most of the mind chatter is gone.

I have been meditating since 1978 but, believe me, it took time to get to a place of quiet in my mind when I first started. Like many of you, I thought I couldn't do it right or I didn't have the time or the proper altar of incense, or space, or chair, or whatever. In truth, though all of those may make meditation more comfortable, none is essential. Except time.

Just like with exercise, you have to take the time. No one is going to give you the time to take care of yourself. It is your responsibility, not anyone else's. Whether your meditation is one minute or one hour, what's important is that you meditate. A patient told me recently she could only sit for a minute. I told her fine! "Sit and focus for one minute, five times a day." During our next visit, she said she was now sitting for five minutes at a time instead of one. This is what I mean by baby steps.

You are not a guru, and you will not be able to clear your mind right away. Like anything, learning to meditate takes time and practice. The key is practice. For one to ten minutes each day, I encourage you to sit down and focus on your breathing. You may want to get up after 10 seconds, call your parents, and suddenly do laundry or clean the bathroom. You will have thoughts, and you will think you are doing it wrong. You aren't. Just bring your focus and attention back to your breathing. Stay seated. The only wrong way to do it is not to do it at all.

If you like, you can light a candle and focus on the flame by putting an image of the flame in your mind, preferably between your eyebrows in the location of your pineal gland in the brain. As mentioned in the chapter on sleep, this gland is where melatonin comes from and has an effect on our circadian rhythm. Ancient and current spiritual leaders believe that it is an organ of universal connection that enables our connection to ALL THAT IS, SOURCE, or GOD.

You might choose to do an Ayurvedic meditation. Place your two middle fingers on the pulse of your right wrist and feel the pulse for two minutes. It's simple and easy to do. Or try a Tibetan singing bowl meditation where you focus on the sound of the bowls. You can find this meditation on YouTube.

It is not necessary to use the word "Ani-Hu" but let me tell you why I use it. *Hu* is a word from Sufism, which is the spiritual aspect of Islam emphasizing the inward search for God. Sufism believes that meditation can bring one closer to God while living and that we do not have to wait until death to experience qualities of or from God. It transcends a particular sect. *Hu* means God. *Ani* is a Sanskrit (classical language of South Asia/India) word that evokes empathy and compassion for self and others.

Hu/man means *God/man*. It's a word that denotes the God connection and consciousness in each of us.

I have found that repeating "Ani-Hu" allows me to go to that place of oneness, compassion, loving, quiet, and peace that I can carry throughout my day. That place enables me to listen, focus and fulfill my purpose here, day to day, by giving me the inner connection to the Source of all things. Meditation brings me into the present moment. There is no past and future, there is only now. And when I find myself not in "now," it is easier to get back to "now" because of my meditation practice. During and after my meditation I experience an energy that is sweet, still, grace-filled, peaceful, forgiving, and compassionate. I recognize there is a place inside of me that is one with All That Is. That place that loves all, forgives all, has compassion for all, and gratitude for the oneness. Meditation allows for being in the present moment, listening. Ideas and awareness come as well during and after meditation. And my concentration is better.

Prayer is talking to God. Meditation is listening to God. I have heard patients say that their pastors warned them against meditating, calling it anti-religious or, even worse, blasphemous. But meditation is non-denominational.

It is not a religion or a philosophy or even a way of being, rather it's meditating on the Light within you. Every religion teaches that having a God consciousness and having a personal relationship with God is essential for well-being. For me, that has been and continues to be true. And God is in all things, everywhere, all the time, including you and me.

We are made in the image of Mother/Father God.

I am not a biblical scholar; however, I am aware of this Bible verse: "And the Word was made flesh, and dwelt among us, full of grace and truth" (John 1:14 KJV). Of course, it is speaking of Jesus Christ, who was God and human. We are all His brothers and sisters, children of God. I believe He came to show us the way to be loving and forgiving of ourselves and others. I believe we are all a part of God, and our flesh is the temple where we can go to seek God and experience forgiveness and loving kindness. Similarly, the Bible says, "Seek ye first the kingdom of heaven (God) and all else will be added unto you" (Matthew 6:33). And in the New King James version in Luke 17:20-21 it says, "The Kingdom of God will not come with observable signs. Nor will people say, 'See here,' or 'See there' it is. For indeed the kingdom of God is within you."

All day I hear my patients talk about the anxiety, depression, fear, and anger they feel because of all that's going on in America and in the world. Those things only add to the day-to-day stresses of family, children, work, relationships, and economic concerns. Meditation is not a panacea, but it is a way to reduce the cascading of stress hormones that begin whenever we hear the news (whether from a friend or the media) of racial discrimination, police brutality, or civil unrest.

The Effects of Meditation

Many of us live with chronic stress. Whether it is about not being able to pay your bills or worrying about having "the conversation" with your son, nephew, or younger brother about what to do when pulled over by the police, the constant pumping of cortisol and adrenaline throughout our bodies affects our genes and increases our predisposition for high blood pressure, diabetes, heart disease, obesity, and cancer—not to mention the damage it does to our mental health.

Stress may be a boss or co-worker who is demeaning and rude. Or the news that is negative and threatening, a friend who is jealous or one who is depressed and anxious, a child on drugs, a parent or sibling with dementia, an ex-partner or current one, your grief, or a simple deadline at work. That mixed with the pressures to "keep up" with everyone else on social media creates constant stress. We need to have something in our lives to stop this bombardment, even if for a moment. We need to have something in our lives to stop the energy of anger, guilt, and resentment that has become part of our daily existence. This energy makes us sick. We must focus on our inner world and let the outer world stop influencing us, again, even for a moment. This is about breaking old habits of thought, feeling, and doing and creating new ones so that you can create a new you in every moment. Those old habits take us out of the present and keep us tied to the past. If there is an event about which you are angry, write about it, without proper English and use curse words if that pleases you, and burn it. Do this as many times as you need to release negative/toxic thoughts and feelings from your past.

I learned early on in a seminar called Insight that energy is just that: energy. We decide how to use it. For example, anxiety and excitement are both energies. You cannot touch those emotions. Pretend you have a coin to go into a jukebox and you can pick any song you like. Anxiety and excitement are the same energy. You can choose anxiety about the job interview or excitement about the job interview. Through meditation, the energy of anxiety will be less familiar to you and therefore will not be the first emotion you choose anymore. You will become aware of options. As with homeopathy, the remedy, which is energy, gets rid of the energy that the body has created in response to some event, thus changing the electromagnetic field (of the immune system) of the person. Moving from unworthiness to increased self-esteem, rage to peace, anxiety to calm, guilt to acceptance, and blame to forgiveness are all possible with meditation as well.

Meditation then can stop so much emotional eating of the comfort food that can be responsible for the dis-eases we experience disproportionately. "Stress affects the same signals as famine does. It turns on the brain pathways that make us crave dense calories—we'll choose high fat, high sweet foods or high salt," says Dr. Elissa Epel, founder of the Center for Obesity Assessment, Study and Treatment at the University of California San Francisco. By calming the central nervous system and our emotions, we are able to have more control over what we eat, when we eat and how much we eat. (Russell, 2014)[81]

Essentially, meditation reduces stress and the releasing of stress hormones like cytokines which create inflammation.[82] Meditation also decreases the risk of heart disease, increases our concentration and attention span, can improve our sleep patterns, help control pain, increases self-awareness, and promotes compassion and positive thinking.[83]

There are many ways to meditate. Choose one and try it for thirty days. If you miss a day, please do not beat yourself up. Just like when a patient misses a day during the detoxification diet, I tell them to go to the next meal and make it even healthier. Similarly, with meditation, we are detoxifying our spirit. Whatever you do, do not judge yourself, just go to the next day and discover what is inside.

I AM LOVED. I AM WELL. I AM GOD'S CHILD.

SALVATION

The act of protecting from harm, risk, loss; preservation or deliverance from harm, risk, loss; the state of being protected from a dire situation.

CHAPTER 10

The Truth as I Know It

When I was five years old, my long-time and dearest friend asked me what I wanted to do when I grew up. Immediately I told her, "I want to save the world." She was nine years older than me and was my brother's friend. She patted me on the head and said, "That's very nice." She was amused. I was serious.

Fast forward, I went to a predominantly White, all-girls high school in Philadelphia. I was continually being called to the principal's office for some bogus event, like having permission to go to the bathroom and then upon my return to class being told I did not have the permission. Hiding in the basement of friends' homes while their parents entertained was customary. I didn't understand then what these events were doing to my self-esteem.

In my sophomore year, whatever strength and dignity remained after the molestation and discriminatory acts was vanquished when my counselor said, "You should not think about college. You should be a domestic worker." I stopped breathing for what seemed like an eternity and I couldn't hear anymore. I only watched her lips move. My grandmother was a domestic worker and her mother a slave. Had my reading, learning, and studying not advanced me beyond their station in life? What would I tell my parents, friends, relatives when it was time to go to college? Words like embarrassment, shame, anguish, and despair do not and cannot describe what I felt that day.

I never spoke a word of this until after I received my PhD in 1976. A reporter for a local newspaper asked to do a story about the one thing for which I thanked my parents most. My response was clear: making me go to college. When my parents first asked where I wanted to go to college, I told them I was going to secretarial school. My father said, "Oh do I need to remind you that the only D you ever received was in typing?" After much conversation and rebuttal, I consented to go to college.

My first year in college was a miserable experience—not just because I was away from home, but also because the school was old and the conditions were at times sub-standard. I ate a tuna cheeseburger and a pack of Twinkies, followed by a Mountain Dew, almost every evening *after* dinner. (Hence the thirty pounds of extra weight I spoke of earlier). I was determined to transfer and stay in school because I loved learning and the process of education. And transfer I did, albeit 30 pounds heavier. By December, I was enrolling in Cheyney University and subsequently graduated second in my class (I was a transfer student). My undergraduate experience came at a time when Dr. Martin Luther King, Jr. and Senator Bobby Kennedy were assassinated. Attending an all-African American university provided a different perspective than what I was used to, a rather reverse racism. And I wasn't accepting of that perspective either.

I entered graduate school specifically to earn a Master's degree in sociology and criminology. In graduate school the dis-ease of racism was ever-present in the classrooms as White professors would tell us the brains of Black people were smaller and this is why we committed more crime, or that Black people *couldn't* learn and this crime was the only avenue for our lives, imprisonment the only consequence. So often I wanted to run out of the classroom and never return. As the only African American in the entire department at the University of Pennsylvania, it seemed as if time had stopped again, and breathing was shallow if at all, as the entire class looked at me to note my response. I was reliving high school and the words of my counselor.

I was studying one day and began to cry. I sobbed for an understanding of the hatred and atrocities in the world and for the inferiority and shame I felt to be *both African American and female.*

Somehow even though I was getting a PhD, I wasn't enough. It wasn't enough. I needed answers that were not of a physical world.

Though raised Episcopalian, I wasn't impressed because we prayed to a pure White Jesus and a God who lived in Heaven. I just did not believe that Jesus could be a White man, given the description in the Bible and because of the part of the world in which he lived. I didn't believe God could be a White man because I looked nothing like that, and we were supposed to be made in the image of God. I was confused.

I sought answers from palm and tarot card readers, psychics, and mystics. My searching finally led me to a spiritual group in California. They spoke of things like how we are all part of God and God is in each one of us. The kingdom of heaven is within and seek ye first the kingdom of heaven and all else will be added unto you. Acceptance, forgiveness (of self for judging others), and loving always in all ways were teachings in seminars I attended.

I felt comfort and some understanding of this world as I heard that we are souls in human form and we have come here to have a physical world experience. And perhaps the things that happen are due to some karma from another lifetime or simply learning for this lifetime. We have come here for spiritual evolution—to know darkness in order to know light in a greater way. Most importantly, we are here to love one another.

With a PhD in hand and some spiritual knowledge, I set out to "save the world," or at least the criminal justice system. I was delusional as that system had already planned to be the end of a pipeline for the underserved and for people of color. It did not take long to see I could not make an impact. Ultimately, I was asked to be a special assistant in President Carter's administration. That is when my life changed.

Dr. D'Adamo told me I should be a naturopath after hearing my story. I told him I was not going back to school for four more years, and every month he would say the same thing: "You should be a naturopathic doctor." And every month, I would say, "Give me some of those bat feathers or whatever you boil in the back room and I am going back to DC." And we would laugh (remember this was 1980 when no one had heard of naturopathic medicine).

I realized All That Is had a different plan for my life when I found myself going back to Howard University where I had been an assistant professor to take pre-requisites for naturopathic school in Seattle, Washington, the cultural opposite of Washington, DC. I was again the only African American in the school, and I cried every day the first year for I had left everything I ever knew as love and home. People asked me if they could touch my hair or if we could be friends because they didn't know any Black people. Thank God for my teachings. I was gracious and relentless in my pursuit of saving the world.

Between my second and third year of school, I took a year off and came home because I was so depressed. I studied with my spiritual group. I learned that *everyone* at some time feels inferior, that abuse was universal and not just in the Black community, that we have so much pain it is difficult to see clearly who we really are: children of God, one people, one race—human. At the end of that year, I didn't just believe in God; I knew God was in everything, everywhere, all the time.

I went back to school after that year because this was/is a calling. Daily I am living my dream of assisting in saving the world one soul at a time. I know All That Is does the work and I am just a vessel. I'm grateful for my dedication to humankind, my determination to let my light shine on the planet when I felt like hiding it, and my discipline to be obedient and faithful to spirit. It was not an easy road.

It doesn't matter where you are in your process toward having a healthier life or how you got where you are. Wherever you are, you can change. Creating good health is not linear and does not happen overnight. None of my Superwomen became suddenly healthy and happy. Nor did I. I'll say it again: good health, or getting to it, is not linear. It took time to change their old habits. The key is they could see the value of the incremental changes, and that encouraged them to stay focused and keep going.

I believe that in life it is helpful to have a vision. And if you are going to have a vision, have a big vision. In addition to treating your hypertension or diabetes, who, what, and how do you want to be in the world? How do you want to live? How do you want to feel? What do you want to look like in two to five years? Decide you are going to change and how you want to change. Write it out. What is your intention? Having an intention makes the methods to get there show up.

Many years ago, I learned in a seminar called Insight how to create a vision board, and I created the life I wanted on that board. I cut out pictures and statements from magazines of the life I wanted and taped them on the poster board. I have pictures of Serena Williams with the words "love your body," Oprah with the words "more than enough," and the words "experience amazing" and "living well" on the board. There are names and pictures of countries where I wanted to travel as well. It was fun doing it and it has been fascinating to see how much of my life is on the board. There were disappointments, for sure–a failed marriage, another that never happened, and financial setbacks during the 2008 market.

But I never stopped faithing, believing, growing, learning, and seeking, and God made a way out of no way. When you were a child and you fell down, you didn't just lie there and say you'll never walk again. You got up and started walking again. With each setback I picked myself up, and I learned that setbacks were God's way of pruning me so I could dig my roots deeper, reach my limbs higher, and experience greater self-love, self-confidence, and a stronger faith in ALL THAT IS/God. I began this book 10 years ago, with an agent who disappeared and reappeared telling me there was no market for this information. Then I had the marriage that never happened, and began taking care of my mother in my home until it was no longer safe. I was in the office five days a week and two Saturdays a month. I was a Superwoman.

Subsequently, I became a Superwoman again. My practice was extremely busy and, after being in the office each day, went to visit with my mother in assisted living and take her organic foods. Not returning home until eight or nine o'clock at night made it a long day. I was happy, blessed, and honored to do it. There was no significant time to write, except perhaps on the weekends. If you have a great relationship with your mother, as I did, or some elder you will at some point be a Superwoman also, if you continue to work and live your life. I continued to exercise on the weekends and on Monday and Wednesday mornings, which were my late days to begin in the office, and one weekend day. Though eating later than I wanted some nights, I still ate well. Sleep was not always before midnight. After my mother passed, I was devastated and didn't write for a year or more. And now this book is in your hands and I am so grateful you chose to read it.

Despite the molestation as a pre-teen, the racism experienced at The Philadelphia High School for Girls, while in graduate school at the University of Pennsylvania and again at Bastyr University, I kept going and striving and believing there was more to life than those experiences. I sought out more mystical and spiritual, if you will, experiences and focused on what I have written in this book in order to learn to love myself more. I believed Spirit had a mission for me which started with naturopathic school.

So here I am wanting you to know and love who you are, however you can do that. It is not easy work and it is so rewarding. When I realized I was a child of All That Is, it changed my life. I am not only African American and female. I am a child of All That Is, God, or whatever your term is that exemplifies loving. And you are as well.

Self-love is a must, it's non-negotiable, but if you don't already have it, you won't cultivate it overnight. That's okay, because the more you do for yourself the more love you have for yourself, and the more love you have for yourself, the more you do for yourself. So, start doing for yourself! Start being and visualizing who you want to be. Remember, self-love is not dependent on how others treat you. It is about how you treat you. It doesn't matter what your parents or relatives said or didn't say about you. Forgive them and move on. You must do whatever is necessary to get rid of beliefs that hold you back.

Start by telling yourself you love yourself. State this while looking at yourself in the mirror, every day, until you believe it. Also write it out. Say it as you wrap your arms around yourself in a big warm hug.

Sometimes, self-love means disconnecting from people who do not have your best interest in mind. They may put you down because they do not feel good about themselves or because they are jealous. It's not about you. It's about them. Those people could be family members or friends. I've disconnected from both at times. The love is still there but I am not going to be in a situation where I am not supported and respected. I am not going to be the topic of gossip and false information while continuing to be in the person's company. I have written about the situations, without any punctuation or inhibitions, many times, if necessary, then burned the pages in order to release whatever hurt or anger the circumstance brought up in me. Subsequently, though I do not choose to be close to them anymore, I not only choose to forgive them, I also forgive myself for judging them as wrong. I choose to have empathy and compassion for them, as I know by their actions, they are troubled. I then write about the act of forgiveness. There are many studies that have shown that resentment, jealousy, and anger all have deleterious effects on one's immune system and thus on one's health. And ask for forgiveness from those you have offended.

I am not a person who spreads gossip, a negative behavior that does not serve anyone. In fact, it weakens you and your spirit. Again, the person who spreads gossip typically has some resentment, envy, or jealousy that affects the mental, emotional, and physical body as well. It's a behavior born of lack of intelligence. Have they nothing else to talk about? Someone once told me, "When you put someone down, all you are doing is putting them down." It doesn't elevate you. Pick yourself up. Do not put anyone down.

Read, go online, and listen to self-improvement podcasts (YouTube, Yale University, Science of Being Well, Insight Seminars, Achieve Today, Emotional Freedom Technique). Depending on how much trauma you've experienced, you may benefit from therapy and of course homeopathy. Seeking therapy doesn't mean you are crazy. It means you have been living in America as an African-American woman with a cultural history of slavery and all of its chains. It means you have come this far doing what you do, and it has gotten you where you are. Be grateful and list those blessings daily in a Gratitude Journal. Also, list one thing you have done well daily. You have survived and persevered. If you are happy where you are, fine. If not, make the decision to take charge of your life and dare to thrive.

Still, take baby steps. Every day do something to change your life. It can be anything from getting up 15 minutes earlier to simply moving your body for 15 minutes or drinking water before breakfast. Make a commitment to yourself. An accountability partner always helps. Ask a neighbor, relative, or a friend to hold you accountable for the goals to which you've committed.

It is true you manifest what you believe, and the universe is here to support you. List your blessings, focus on them, and be grateful now. Don't wait until you get that degree or job or start your business or write a book to be grateful. Be grateful now. Act as if it has already happened. Design your future the way you want it. Write the story of who you are one year from now; three years from now; five years from now. What is your level of health? What do you look like? What are you doing? Where are you living? What kind of work are you doing? What is your income? Play with your future. See it in your mind. Feel it in your body.

Use your imagination and feel the way it would feel if your goals were accomplished and were in existence now. Do this daily. Write it down. God loves and supports you and God has to know what you want. You have to meet God halfway by moving in the direction of what you say you want. I tell my patients all the time, if you want to buy a car you have to go online or go to the car lot. The car is not going to come crashing through your living room window.

God did not intend for you to be ill, upset, and depressed all the time. God did not put you here in this thing called life to dump you and never assist you. Life is precious and so are you. Please take care of yourself. The planet needs you. Do something daily that gives you strength spiritually, mentally, emotionally, and physically.

Again, good health takes time. It is not linear. Letitia said to me recently, "It's been awesome, feeling better. No stomach issues or other issues. It takes some effort and reflection at first but it is possible to be done. I'm not slipping into old habits now, and I don't let stuff stress me or worry me, especially my children. I have done my best with the resources I had."

Your piece of the puzzle has to be present for someone else's piece to fit. We are interconnected. I know it is difficult to conceive, especially today in this country, and we are one people, one race—the human race. In *The Tibetan Book of Living and Dying*, Sogyal Rinpoche says, "True spirituality also is to be aware that if we are interdependent with everything and everyone else, even our smallest, least significant thought, word, and action have real consequences throughout the universe. Everything is inextricably interrelated: We come to realize we are responsible for everything we do, say or think, responsible in fact for ourselves…"

Bob Doyle, one of the participants in the documentary "The Secret", stated simply, "Create a new life from scratch." Below I share more of the Truth as I know it:

- Realize you are more than enough.
- Be responsible for what you put in your body, mind, and soul. You are the temple where God resides.
- Take time to go inside and explore. There is so much outside yourself that distracts you and gives you false messages. Go inside.
- No one is responsible for your joy or lack thereof. That is between you and your God. The kingdom of heaven is within. Go there.

- How can you have more peace? Stop being at war with yourself and others.
- Now is the moment that never ends.
- Progression is the expansion of happiness and compassion.
- Laugh more today than yesterday.
- Create new experiences.
- Practice who you want to be and who you are becoming.
- The fastest way to get what you want is to say "no" to what you don't want.
- "No" is a whole sentence.
- Decide what is going to change and make that happen, even if it is one thing.
- Thoughts are powerful and negative thoughts in particular are addictive, habitual, and stressful. Start having positive thoughts.
- Forgive yourself for judging yourself and others as wrong.
- Be faithful. It is easy to be faithful when things are going great. Faith is believing that things are perfect even when they are not great.
- Everything is perfect, especially when you do not like it.
- Acceptance is the first law of Spirit—accept all of you and commit to change.
- Are you a Superwoman? There always is and always will be something to do for someone else. Do something for yourself today.
- As Serena Williams says, "Never give up."
- As Mary Lou Sullivan said, "Know that everything is going to be alright."

I AM LOVED.　I AM WELL.　I AM GOD'S CHILD.

EPILOGUE

Bring what has worked for you into the now and move forward:

F = Faithing, forgiveness
O = Organic–natural life or living matter
R = Renew self, reward self, recreate self through daily ritual
W = Water, winner, wisdom (inner)
A = Ask for what you want, affirmation
R = Rejoice, give thanks
D = Divinity/God's child

And celebrate:

C = Choice, create your life day to day moment to moment
E = Empower yourself
L = Love yourself
E = Easy–be gentle with yourself
B = Be brave and bold
R = Rest and rejuvenate
A = Acceptance
T = Tell your truth
E = Energy is available to you when making life changes

We are super women. We are bold, bright, beautiful, daring, caring, charitable, creative, nurturing, faithful, strong, delicate, fearless, powerful, sensitive, loving, kind, formidable, vulnerable, and gracious. Let us be a part of the cycle of giving and receiving to and from ourselves, such that we know WELLNESS is but one more example of God's Grace.

God bless us all.

BIOGRAPHY

In 1976, Andrea Sullivan was the first African American to receive a PhD from the University of Pennsylvania in Sociology/Criminology. She taught at Howard University, American University, and the University of Maryland, and was subsequently appointed Assistant Director of the Administration of Justice for the National Urban League in New York City. She later worked as a Special Assistant for Urban Policy to Patricia Roberts Harris, the US Secretary of Housing and Urban Development (HUD) during the Carter administration.

Dr. Sullivan received an ND (Doctor of Naturopathic Medicine degree) from Bastyr University in Seattle, Washington in 1986—the first African American woman to graduate from that university. After completing the four-year accredited program, Dr. Sullivan also took advanced courses in homeopathic medicine in the United States, India, and Europe. She continues to study with homeopathic physicians from Mumbai, India and is a Diplomate with the Homeopathic Academy of Naturopathic Physicians.

Dr. Sullivan is a founding member of the American Association of Naturopathic Physicians and served as president of the D.C. Association of Naturopathic Physicians for eight years. In 2007, she was also appointed by the mayor of the nation's capital to serve as chairperson of the Naturopathic Medical Board for the District of Columbia, after having served on the Board of Medicine for five years. Most recently, Dr. Sullivan received an Honorary Doctor of Science degree from Sonoran University of Health Sciences in Tempe, Arizona. She has a private practice in Washington, D.C.

Excerpts from her successful first book, *A Path to Healing: A Guide to Wellness for Body, Mind, and Soul* (Doubleday 1998), appeared in *Essence Magazine* in July 1998, followed by several feature stories on Dr. Sullivan over the following years. Dr. Sullivan is also a contributing writer to *Prevention, Essence, Ebony, Huffington Post, Heart and Soul,* and *Health Quest* publications.

As of November 2021, she became a member of the International Women's Forum, an invitation–only network connecting women leaders across every professional sector with the common mission of advancing women's leadership and championing equality around the world. Currently IWF is composed of over 7,500 preeminent women leaders in 33 countries and 74 local forums.

Dr. Sullivan is frequently a guest on radio and major network television, The Shift Network, and podcasts, and travels throughout the country and Canada to lecture on naturopathic medicine and wellness.

BIBLIOGRAPHY

Ahmad, U. A. (2018, July 27). Antihyperlipidemic efficacy of aqueous extract of Stevia rebaudiana Bertoni in albino rats. *Lipids in Health and Disease, 17*(1), 175.

AJ, L. (2009, May). Should dairy be recommended as part of a healthy vegetarian diet? *Am J Clin Nutrition, 89*(5), 1638S-1642S.

An R, M. J. (2016, October 29). Plain water consumption in relation to energy intake and diet quality among US adults, 2005-2012. *J Hum Nutr Diet, 5*, 624-32.

Anton SD, M. C. (2010, August). Effects of stevia, aspartame, and sucrose on food intake, satiety, and postprandial glucose and insulin levels. *Appetite, 55*(1), 37-43.

Aune D, N. R. (2015, January). Dairy products, calcium, and prostate cancer risk: a systematic review and meta-analysis of cohort studies. *American Journal Clinical Nutrition, 101*(1), 87-117.

Banister CE, M. A. (2015, January 1). Disparity in the persistence of high-risk human papillomavirus genotypes between African American and European American women of college age. *J Infect Dis, 211*(1), 100-8.

Bar-Or O, D. R. (1985). Voluntary Hypohydration in 10–12-year-old boys. *J. Applied Physiology* (40), 104-108.

Barry M Popkin, K. E. (2010, August 1). Water, hydration, and health. *Nutrition Reviews, 68*(8), 439–458.

Batmanghelidj, F. (1992). *our body's many cries for water: Don't treat thirst with medications: body thirst signals and damages of chronic dehydration are explained: a preventive and self-education manual for those who prefer to adhere to the logic of the natural and the simple.* Falls Church, VA, USA: Global Health Solutions.

Bieiweis, B. B. (2020, August 3). *The Basic Facts About Women in Poverty.* Retrieved from https://www.americanprogress.org/article/basic-facts-women-poverty/#:~:text=Quick%20facts%20about%20women%20living,of%20the%20federal%20poverty%20line.

Black and White. (2018). *National Geographic.*

Cian C, B. P. (2001). Effects of fluid ingestion on cognitive function after heat stress or exercise induced dehydration. *International Journal of Psychophysiology, 41,* 243-45.

Cooper, A. J. (1892). *A Voice from the South.* Xenia, Ohio, USA: The Aldine Printing House.

Corbett, H. (2020, August 13). *Why Black Women's Equal Pay Day 2020 Is So Important.* Retrieved July 2022, from www.forbes.com: https://www.forbes.com/sites/hollycorbett/2020/08/13/why-black-womens-equal-pay-day-2020-is-so-important/?sh=6b31265b21c2

Craig, M. (2002). *Ain't I a Beauty Queen?: Black Women, Beauty, and the Politics of Race.* USA: Oxford University Press.

Culp KR, W. B. (2004, Aug). Bioelectrical impedance analysis and other hydration parameters as risk factors for delirium in rural nursing home residents. *J Gerontol A Biol Sci Med Sci., 59*(8), 813-7.

D Anci KE, V. A. (2009). Voluntary dehydration a cognitive performance in trained college athletes. *Precept Mot Skills, 109,* 251-269.

Diabetes and African Americans. (2021, 3 1). Retrieved from Office of Minority Health (OMH) at the U.S. Department of Health and Human Services: https://minorityhealth.hhs.gov/omh/browse.aspx?lvl=4&lvlid=18

DiNicolantonio JJ, O. J. (2018, July). Sugar addiction: is it real? A narrative review. *Br J Sports Medicine, 52*(14), 910-913.

Dornas WC, d. L. (2019, July 15). Health implications of high-fructose intake and current research. *The Journal of Physiology, 597*(14), 3561-3571.

Freedman, R. B. (2005). *Skinny Bitch: A No-Nonsense, Tough-Love Guide for Savvy Girls Who Want to Stop Eating Crap and Start Looking Fabulous.* Running Press Adult.

Geronimus, A. T. (1992, Summer). The weathering hypothesis and the health of African -American women and Infants: evidence and speculations. *Ethnicity and Disease, 2* (3), 207-220.

Howell, E. (2018, June). Reducing Disparities in Severe Maternal Morbidity and Mortality. *Clin Obstet Gynecol, 61*(2), 387-399.

Kimball, R. (2020). *Who Rules?: Sovereignty, Nationalism, and the Fate of Freedom in the Twenty-First Century.* Encounter Books.

Knisely, S. (2017, March 27). *The 1920s Women Who Fought For the Right to Travel Under Their Own Names.* Retrieved from Atlas Obscura: https://www.atlasobscura.com/articles/us-passport-history-women#:~:text=%E2%80%9CThe%20Lucy%20Stone%20League%20saw,Ruth%20Hale%2C%20and%20Jane%20Grant.

Knut Dahl-Jørgensen, G. J. (1991, November 1). Relationship Between Cows' Milk Consumption and Incidence of IDDM in Childhood. *Diabetes Care, 14*(11), 1081–1083.

Lust, B. (1937). *Naturopath and Herald of Health* (Vol. 22).

M.D., G. C. (2000). *Conscious Eating.* North Atlantic Books.

Malosse D, P. H. (1992). Correlation between milk and dairy product consumption and multiple sclerosis prevalence: a worldwide study. *Neuroepidemiology, 11*(4-6), 304-12.

Michals, D. (2015). *Sojourner Truth.* Retrieved from National Women's

History Museum: https://www.womenshistory.org/education-resources/biographies/sojourner-truth

Mitchell, P. W. (2018, October 4). The fault in his seeds: Lost notes to the case of bias in Samuel George Morton's cranial race science. *PLOS Biology, 16*(10).

Mullings, L. (2002, June 28). The Sojourner Syndrome: Race, Class, and Gender in Health and Illness. *Voices* (6), 32-36.

Obesity and African Americans. (2019). Retrieved May 2022, from U.S. Department of Health and Human Services (HHS): https://minorityhealth.hhs.gov/omh/browse.aspx?lvl=4&lvlid=25

Okamoto-Mizuno, K. M. (2012, May 31). Effects of Thermal Environment on Sleep and Circadian Rhythm. *Journal of Physiological Anthropology, 31*(14).

Ostchega Y, F. C. (2020, April). Hypertension Prevalence Among Adults Aged 18 and Over: United States, 2017-2018. *NCHS Data Brief* (364), 1-8.

Quanhe Yang, P., Zefeng Zhang, M. P., Edward W. Gregg, P., & al, e. (2014). Added Sugar Intake and Cardiovascular Diseases Mortality Among US Adults. *JAMA Intern Medicine, 174*(4), 516-524.

Richardson, L. C., Henley, S. J., Miller, J. W., Massetti, G., & Thomas, C. C. (2016). Patterns and trends in age-specific black-white differences in breast cancer incidence and mortality - United States, 1999-2014. *Morbidity and Mortality Weekly Report, 65*(40), 1093-1098.

Rona RJ, K. T. (2007, September). The prevalence of food allergy: a meta-analysis. *J Allergy Clin Immunology, 120*(3), 638-46.

Russell, S. (2014). *Success Through Stillness.* Avery.

Sleep. (2020, October). *National Geographic*, p. 26. Retrieved from

National Geographic.

Suhr JA, H. J. (2004). The relation of hydration status to cognitive performance in healthy older adults. *International Journal of Psychophysiology, 53*, 121-125.

Sullivan, A. (1999). *A Path to Healing: A Guide to Wellness for Body, Mind, and Soul.* Main Street Books.

Survey, L. F. (2022, July 08). *Bureau of Labor Statistics.* Retrieved from Unemployment rates by age, sex, race, and Hispanic or Latino ethnicity: https://www.bls.gov/web/empsit/cpsee_e16.htm

The Charleston Medical Journal and Review. (1852). Charleston S.C., Burges & James.

The Race Issue. (2018, March). *National Geographic.* Retrieved from National Geographic: https://www.nationalgeographic.com/magazine/issue/april-2018

USHistory.org. (n.d.).

Villarosa, L. (1994). *Body & soul: The Black women's guide to physical health and emotional well-being.*

Villarosa, L. (2022). *Under the Skin.* Doubleday.

Voyer P, R. S. (2009, May). Predisposing factors associated with delirium among demented long term care residents. *Clinical Nutrition Research, 18*(2), 153-71.

Weber KS, S. M. (2018, June 15). Habitual Fructose Intake Relates to Insulin Sensitivity and Fatty Liver Index in Recent-Onset Type 2 Diabetes Patients and Individuals without Diabetes. *Nutrients, 10*(6), 774.

Williams, R. (2009, June). Cardiovascular disease in African American women: a health care disparities issue. *J Natl Med Assoc., 101*(6), 536-40.

Winkler, K. J. (n.d.). The Life of the Legendary Sojourner Truth: A New Biography Explores the Facts and Fictions. *The Chronicle of*

Higher Education, 43(3).

Women's Rights: National Historical Park. (2022, June 11). Retrieved from USHistory.org: http://npshistory.com/publications/wori/index.htm

Woods-Giscombé, C. (2010, May). Superwoman schema: African American women's views on stress, strength, and health. *Qual Health Res., 20*(5), 668-683.

ENDNOTES

1. (Mullings, 2002)
2. https://www.norhtcarolinahealthnews.org/202`1/05/24/black-patients-covid-symptoms-more-often-diseissed-downplayed/
3. https://.kffhealthnews.org/news/covid-19-treatment-racial-income-health-disparities/
4. (Ostchega Y, 2020)
5. (Richardson, Henley, Miller, Massetti, & Thomas, 2016)
6. (Diabetes and African Americans, 2021)
7. (Banister CE, 2015)
8. (Kimball, 2020)
9. https://.doi.org/10.1016/50027-9684(15)30938-X
10. (Williams, 2009)
11. https://www.ncbi.nlm.nih.gov/pmc/articles/PMC7583499
12. (Survey, 2022)
13. (Corbett, 2020)
14. (Bieiweis, 2020)
15. https://doi.org/10.1016/j.cities.2023.104297
16. (Michals, 2015)
17. (Craig, 2002)
18. (Winkler)
19. https://www.brookings.edu. The history of women's work and wages by Janet Yellen. May 2023
20. (Knisely, 2017)
21. (Cooper, 1892)
22. (Woods-Giscombé, 2010)

23 (Geronimus, 1992)

24 (Howell, 2018)

25 (Obesity and African Americans, 2019)

26 (Villarosa L. , 1994)

27 https:www.washingtonpost.com/politics/2023/07/22/desantis-slavery-curriculum

28 en.wikipedia.org/wiki/Slavery_in_the_colonial_history_of_the_United_States

29 (Mitchell, 2018)

30 (Mitchell, 2018)

31 (The Race Issue, 2018)

32 https://www.mayoclinic.org/drugs-supplements/betacarotene-oral-route/precautions/drg-20066795

33 Lete I. AllueJ. The Effectiveness of Ginger in the Prevention of Nausea and Vomiting during Pregnancy and Chemotherapy. Integr Med Insights 2016 Mar 31:11:11-7. doi:10.4137/IMI.S36273. PMID: 27053918; PMCID: PMC4818

34 https:www.mayoclinic.org/diseases-conditions/cancer/expert-answers/curcumin/faq-20057858#:~:twxt=it's%20being%20exploired%20as%20a,from%20damage%20by%20radiation

35 Peng Y, Ao M, Dong B, Jiang Y, Yu L, Chen Z, Hu C, Xu R. Anti-Inflammatory Effects of Curcumin in the Inflammatory Diseases: Status, Limitations and Countermeasures. Drug Des Devel Ther. 2021 Nov 2;15:4503-4525. doi: 10.2147/DDDT.S327378. PMID: 34754179; PMCID: PMC8572027.

36 https://www.webmd.com/diet/health-benefits-ashwagandha#:~:text=High%20and%20chronic%20stress%20levels,blood%20pressure%20and%20heart%20rate

37 Mishra LC, Singh BB, Dagenais S. Scientific basis for the therapeutic use of Withania somnifera(ashwagandha): a review. Altern Med Rev. 2000 Aug;5(4):334-46. PMID: 10956379.

38 Wankhede S, Langade D, Joshi K, Sinha SR, Bhattacharyya S. Examining the effect of Withania somnifera supplementation on muscle strength and recovery: a randomized controlled trial. J Int Soc Sports Nutr. 2015 Nov 25;12:43. doi: 10.1186/s12970-015-0104-9. PMID: 26609282; PMCID: PMC4658772.

39 Ried K. Garlic lowers blood pressure in hypertensive subjects, improves arterial stiffness and gut microbiota: A review and meta-analysis. Exp Ther Med. 2020 Feb;19(2):1472-1478. doi: 10.3892/etm.2019.8374. Epub 2019 Dec 27. PMID: 32010325; PMCID: PMC6966103.

40 Sharma V, Sharma A, Kansal L. The effect of oral administration of Allium sativum extracts on lead nitrate induced toxicity in male mice. Food Chem Toxicol. 2010 Mar;48(3):928-36. doi: 10.1016/j.fct.2010.01.002. Epub 2010 Jan 12. PMID: 20060875.

41 https://doi.org/10.33545/26174693.2018.v2.i1a.113

42 (Sullivan, 1999)

43 (Lust, 1937)

44 https://perspectivesofchange.hms.harvard.edu/node/99

45 (Villarosa L. , 2022)

46 https://www.betterup.com

47 Zhang Y, Coca A, Casa DJ, Antonio J, Green JM, Bishop PA. Caffeine and diuresis during rest and exercise: A meta-analysis. J Sci Med Sport. 2015 Sep;18(5):569-74. doi: 10.1016/j.jsams.2014.07.017. Epub 2014 Aug 9. PMID: 25154702; PMCID: PMC4725310.

48 Czarnecka K, Pilarz A, Rogut A, Maj P, Szymańska J, Olejnik Ł, Szymański P. Aspartame-True or False? Narrative Review

of Safety Analysis of General Use in Products. Nutrients. 2021 Jun 7;13(6):1957. doi: 10.3390/nu13061957. PMID: 34200310; PMCID: PMC8227014.

49 (An R, 2016)

50 (Bar-Or O, 1985)

51 (D Anci KE, 2009)

52 (Suhr JA, 2004)

53 (Cian C, 2001)

54 (Culp KR, 2004)

55 (Voyer P, 2009)

56 (Batmanghelidj, 1992)

57 (DiNicolantonio JJ, 2018)

58 (Quanhe Yang, Zefeng Zhang, Edward W. Gregg, & al, 2014)

59 (Weber KS, 2018)

60 (Dornas WC, 2019)

61 Regnat K, Mach RL, Mach-Aigner AR. Erythritol as sweetener-wherefrom and whereto? Appl Microbiol Biotechnol. 2018 Jan;102(2):587-595. doi: 10.1007/s00253-017-8654-1. Epub 2017 Dec 1. PMID: 29196787; PMCID: PMC5756564.

62 https://www.nih.gov/news-events/nih-research-matters/erythritol-cardiovascular-events#:~:text=Higher%20blood%20levels%20of%20the,term%20risks%20for%20cardiovascular%20health.

63 https://www.medicalnewstoday.com/articles/monk-fruit-benefits#benefits

64 (Freedman, 2005)

65 (Aune D, 2015)

66 (DiNicolantonio JJ, 2018)

67 (Knut Dahl-Jørgensen, 1991)

68 (Malosse D, 1992)

69 (Rona RJ, 2007)

70 https://www.betterhealth.vic.gov.au

71 https://doi.org/10.1136/bmj.g6015

72 Hilliard CB. High osteoporosis risk among East Africans linked to lactase persistence genotype. Bonekey Rep. 2016 Jun 29;5:803. doi: 10.1038/bonekey.2016.30. PMID: 27408710; PMCID: PMC4926535.

73 https://www.healthline.com by What's the pH of Milk and Does It Matter for Your Body by Noreen Iftikhar,MD June 18, 2018

74 https://www.sleepfoundation.org/bedroom

75 https://www.sleepfoundation.org/bedroom-environment/blue-light

76 https://pubmed.ncbi.nlm.nih.gov/15583226/ and https://pubmed.ncbi.nlm.nih.gov/26612385

77 https://doi.org/10.1038/s41598-020-65086-x

78 https://www.tandfonline.com/doi/full/10.1080/13548506.2019.1612075

79 https://dx.doi.org/10.5888/pcd17.190424

80 (Sleep, 2020)

81 (Russell, 2014)

82 https://doi.org/10.1016/j.cpnec.2021.100037

83 https://doi.org/10.1016/j.cpnec.2021.100037

www.ingramcontent.com/pod-product-compliance
Lightning Source LLC
LaVergne TN
LVHW041949070526
838199LV00051BA/2962